p. 67 Good pt.

p. 291 ACE questionn

p. 297 Expanded Trauma question.

p. 309 The Resiliency Ques.

GENERATIONS DEEP

Unmasking Inherited Dysfunction and Trauma to Rewrite Our Stories Through Faith and Therapy

To Jason - a friend in Christ and fellow Cardinals fan!

GINA BIRKEMEIER, MAC, LPC

Gina Birkemeier, LPC

Published by Out Loud Publishing

ISBN: 978-1-7329545-2-6 (paperback)

Cover Design: Sharisse Coulter Designs
Developmental Edits: Book Coaching Works
Interior Design: Mind the Margins

First paperback edition.

Printed in the USA.

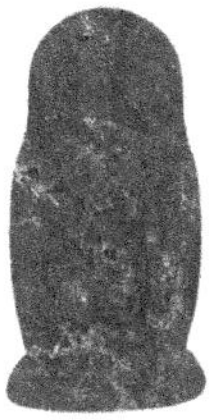

"I did then what I knew how to do.
Now that I know better, I do better."

MAYA ANGELOU

To My Children, those born to me and those gifted in marriage:
I'm sorry I didn't know sooner. Thank you for forgiving me.

To My Husband: You are my best corrective experience.

To My Savior: You make all things new.

TABLE OF CONTENTS

An Introduction....................1

Prologue....................7

What We Pass On....................7

PART ONE – Things to Consider While Reading *Generations Deep*....................9

Chapter 1: Guidance for This Journey....................11

How to Use This Book....................14

PART TWO – Generations Past: Patterns Set in Motion....................17

Chapter 2: Coming to America....................21

A Whole New World....................22

Angelo and Lucia....................23

Restless Hearts....................25

A New Family....................28

Chapter 3: Blood Is Thicker Than Water....................33

Marie (and Charlie)....................34

A Bond Not Easily Broken....................37

A Missing Piece....................38

Chapter 4: Patterns Continue into Modern Times....................41

Marie and Cathy....................41

Chapter 5: Pattern Turns Deadly....................47

Marie's Goodbye....................47

Finding Charlie....................48

Cathy....................49

PART THREE – In My Life: Patterns and Pain Repeating....................53

Chapter 6: My Birth and Adoption Story....................55

The Original Version of the Story....................55

Adopted—Twice....................58

Unsure of My Place....................60

Chapter 7: Repair or Inherit....65

The Problems with Secrets and Shame....65

A Striking Resemblance....67

More on Chaos....68

Hope for Judy....73

Hope Lost....75

Breaking a Child's Heart....76

Chapter 8: Hoping for Hope....81

A Refuge Lost....81

Finding Connection....84

Somehow, You Just Know....87

Ernie Had a Secret Too....88

Meeting Cathy Again....92

Chapter 9: Wanting It to Work....97

Auditioning for Family....97

Chapter 10: A Darker Spiral....103

The Last of Innocence Lost....103

Just Like the Big Kids....108

Chapter 11: Deepening Distrust....111

Moving Out....111

A Final Blow to Innocence....116

Failed Attempt to Get Help....124

Chapter 12: A Science Break....129

Missing Time and the Body's Response....129

Science Meets Scripture: Transgenerational Epigenetic Inheritance....131

Given Up Twice–Revisited....136

Chapter 13: Adulthood....143

Too Many Jagged Little Pills....143

Deepest Regrets and Hidden Privilege....146

Chapter 14: A Glimpse of God 151
Jesus Freaks *151*
Turning Tides on a Shifting Sea *154*
You Can't Fix Decades Overnight *155*
Blessings in Disguise *157*

PART FOUR – Finding Father **163**
Chapter 15: Missing Pieces 165
Cathy's Gift *165*
Risking Wounds *168*
Cheryl: A Re-Introduction *173*
A Hard Day's Night *176*
Meet My Husband *180*
Letting Tom Help *183*
Close to Home *184*
Reinforcements *186*
A Break in the Case *188*
Meeting Dean *196*

Chapter 16: The Best Gift 205
Happy Birthday to Me *205*

Chapter 17: He Can Be Trusted 215
Sometimes You Just Know It's a God Thing *215*

PART FIVE – Healing Present and Past **219**
Chapter 18: Unexpected Places of Healing 221
The Good with the Bad *221*
A Timely Experience *226*
There's Always More to the Story *230*

lots of good advice
"Healing doesn't happen in a straight line"

PART SIX – Emotionally Corrective Experiences **233**
Chapter 19: Turning Toward Healing 235
What Helps Us Heal *235*
Healing Wounds *236*

PART SEVEN – Jesus and A Therapist **257**

Chapter 20: Mental Health in Christian Circles 259

The Case for Holistic Healing *259*

Struggling Despite Our Faith .... *262* good perspective

Changing Our Thoughts *264*

PART EIGHT – A Word from Fellow Travelers **269**

Chapter 21: Encouragement and Questions 271

Questions and Encouragements from My Fellow Travelers ... *274*

Shining a Light *278*

PART NINE – Your Turn **285**

Chapter 22: Exploring and Expanding Your Journey 287

Expanding Your Perspective *288*

Adverse Childhood Experience (ACE) Questionnaire 291

Expanding Your Perspective (A Little More) *292*

The Expanded Trauma Perspective Questionnaire 297

Their Turn *303*

Pain Outside the Family *306*

Resiliency Can Be Generational Too *306*

The Resilience Questionnaire 309

PART TEN – Therapy Things **313**

Chapter 23 : Thoughts on (Some) Therapies that Help 315

Thoughts on Therapeutic Approaches *316*

Therapeutic Favorites (So Far) *319*

Finding the Right Counselor *331*

The Faith and Science of Generational Impact *334*

Endings and Beginnings *335*

PART ELEVEN – Epilogue **337**

It Takes a Village *341*

Resource Page **345**

Generations/Family Relationships Chart **347**

An Introduction

Greetings, New Friend,

Want to know a secret?

The book you now hold in your hands is not the book I intended to write. True, I wanted to write a book that would be helpful to people on their journey of discovery and healing. But I thought I could do that by writing something that merely touched my story, rather than telling it in detail. My hope was to offer help while remaining *slightly* detached. I should have known better.

"Detached" has never been my style.

So, after several starts and stops, and encounters with many individuals working tirelessly to make sense of their own stories, I knew if this book had any hope of achieving its goal, it would need to be written in the way it was *asking* to be written. I knew I needed to tell my story.

Lots of risk comes with saying "yes" to putting your story out there, especially when the story involves the generations before you and the ones after. I had to say "no" to some things in order to stay true to the course set before me, including what others might think of the finished product.

My hope is that the book you now hold offers enough faith, therapy and science to provide enough hope and encouragement to explore your own story and the story of those who went before you.

I know the idea of an expedition like this can be challenging. It is difficult to think about the past generations. We prefer to look at the beautiful things they left with us, like an inherited talent or trait, or one of Nana's lovely heirlooms, usually to the exclusion of what has been passed down that might be less beautiful.

While the pull to exclude is understandable, those exclusions can hold consequences for us, like the potential to repeat the mistakes from previous generations and continue unhealthy cycles.

The truth is, if we really want to respect the generations gone by, we must learn from them, and if possible, grow beyond them. It might not be easy, but it is possible to acknowledge and accept both the good things we have inherited and the not-so-good things at the same time. We do not need to choose one or the other. In fact, being able to hold the two truths in tension is one of the healthiest things we can learn to do. The ability to hold seemingly conflicting emotions "in tension" helps us avoid the toxic trap of feeling we must choose, which can feel invalidating. Ideas like "this is hard *and* I can do this" or "this is painful *and* I'm comforted by those supporting me" are just a couple examples. This is a skill we can learn *and* pass on to others.

And *that* is something of which Nana would be proud.

Before we get too deep in my story, let me say that I realize there are a lot of stories out there, and I value your decision to read mine. We are on this journey together, and I promise to provide you with valuable insights and information along the way based on my professional experience and personal story.

A little bit of background: For a very long time, I have been somewhat of a self-help groupie, combined with a deep thirst for the spiritual. I began therapy (both in and outside of my faith) some 25 years ago.

Although my academic career was less than traditional, I fell in love with all things psychological in undergrad. The more family systems were discussed, the more of a pull I felt to really grasp the story of generations before me. Sometimes I would sit in class and think about my own trauma and the mistakes I had made out of my own pain, and find myself asking *"How did I get here?"* I was not ready to do the deeper work at that time. That would come much later and after much therapy *and* much Jesus. Throughout the years I would find myself attempting to fill in all the blanks that come with being adopted, yet still being raised within the same biological family system, which is a big part of the story you will be reading.

The more healing I experienced, the more I knew I wanted to help others find their own healing. This has taken a variety of shapes over the years, beginning in ministry and pastoral counseling and care roles. Still, there was more ground to cover in my personal healing before I could expand that work.

Over the years, I have worked in licensed counseling and pastoral care roles in churches, nonprofits and counseling centers. In all of those roles, time and time again, I would find myself coming back to the work of unearthing generational patterns with my clients and in my own life. And time after time new awareness, understanding and healing would result, along with grace for ourselves and often for those who had gone before us.

Later in my career, I sat under the mentorship of Dr. Leonard Matheson, a neurorehabilitation psychologist who works from a redemptive world view, rooted in his belief in God. While his contribution to my education and ability to counsel is immeasurable, so is the added healing I experienced as a result of that relationship. In my work with him, I

continued to see a pervasive pattern of generational experiences contributing to the *dis-ease* of my clients, as well as my own.

The more I learned about my family and the more I worked with clients uncovering information about their own familial relations, the more this idea of patterns repeating would surface. I knew that biblically and scientifically; this whole generational thing was really a *thing!* Terms like "intergenerational trauma" and "generational wounds" appeared more and more on the playing field, emboldening my work with clients and even in my own life.

Then, several years ago, I was introduced to terms like "behavioral epigenetics," and something called Transgenerational Epigenetic Inheritance. There is a great deal yet to be discovered in both of these scientific areas, but the research thus far has been instrumental in pressing me forward to write the book you now hold in your hands. In short, these areas of science give us some solid data to support the idea that what we inherit matters, perhaps more than we realize. Not in a "doomed to repeat history" sort of way, but in a way that gives us more insight into what it is we might need to deconstruct in our story in order to build the heathy, hope-filled life God intended for us to live.

It was in understanding patterns from my own family and the consequences not only of my own trauma, but of theirs, that I was able to see the contributing factors in the "false narrative" that guided my life to that point—this false narrative that had been written, in part, before I even took my first breath.

And so, it is with all of us.

In those generations that came before us, our understanding of ourselves, others, the world around us and even God is informed from this place. At some point, those ideas and beliefs become deeply ingrained, even solidified, by our experiences, interactions with caregivers and the

messages we absorb from those around us—whether implicit or explicit; covert or overt. Eventually we adopt those beliefs as our own and adapt our way of living to conform **and confirm** them. Sadly, that's not always a good thing.

Sometimes it takes a Divine intervention for us to realize the story we are living is not the one we have been created for. That was true for me.

So, as we journey together through the coming pages, as you read my story and consider your own, it is my hope that you see me as your "companion in the battle." There is a reason *"Breaking cycles. Slaying shame. Finding freedom."* can be found everywhere in my writing, speaking and web presence. It is more than a kitschy phrase.

It is my battle cry.

And it is my passion and mission to help make it yours, too. So, I will armor up, link arms and stand with you in the battle to help you slay shame. Anytime. Anywhere. That is a promise.

I hope that my story emboldens you to explore your story. And I hope you discover places of understanding and opportunities to disrupt patterns of belief and behavior that stem from a false narrative. You may just realize, *the truth of what you believe about yourself isn't true at all. And that can set you free to write a new story—the one intended for you.*

Prologue

WHAT WE PASS ON

> "The sins of the father are visited upon future generations..."
> EXODUS 34:7

Oh, how I used to hate this verse. I once had a client tell me that she hated it, too. It made her think of an-impossible-to-please, vengeful god. A god she wanted no part of. I completely understood, because for a big part of my life, I agreed with her.

But then one day, a different perspective on this controversial verse presented itself to me. One that I shared with my client. It's one I would like to share with you, too.

What if this verse is not some warning of wrath from a vengeful, punitive deity? What if this verse is not talking about something God does *to* us, but rather something we do to ourselves—and to each other?

What if this verse is *actually* a compassionate, albeit cryptic, warning? Perhaps it is a rallying cry to get us to show up and own our crap; to heal and to grow, and to set future generations up to do the same. What

if this verse is a plea from on High to recognize our choices can set off ripple effects that are far beyond our understanding and that our choices influence the future beyond what we are able to recognize in the tangible, relational realms.

And what if this ominous, poetic warning is really pointing us toward something much more scientific and even *holistic*? What if it's a prooftext that we are incapable of living compartmentalized lives—that every part of us is inextricably connected to the other, not only within our own lives, but in all the lives that lead up to our existence? What if the ripples set in motion by those who have gone before us cast destructive waves upon the present and have potential to reach into future generations, unless there is some intervention?

Could it be that what we perceive as a threat in this verse is actually a reminder that we are integrated beings; the spiritual impacts the emotional impacts the physical impacts the mental impacts the spiritual, beginning long before we took our first breath?

Perhaps this message is the ultimate expression of loving guidance. An Omniscient warning to pay attention to more than just the present. Because the reality is that what came before us will play out in the here-and-now. Maybe this warning is telling us to take caution with how we live and whether we choose to heal, because the One giving the warning knows it will impact not only us, but also those who come after us, and those who come after them... to the third and fourth generations.

If, like me, you are willing to accept this idea, then keep it with you as you read through my story. Remember it as we visit some tough places. It is the call to action. The call of Hope.

PART ONE

Things to Consider While Reading *Generations Deep*

CHAPTER 1 Guidance for This Journey

As I share my story, I will help you make sense of what may occasionally feel incohesive in the timeline—something I can only do from this side of healing. The research is clear: when there is trauma, neglect and/or pervasive chaos in childhood, or excessive use of substances at a young age, there are often gaps and less-than-linear recollections of our history. Often, it is the brain's attempt at protecting us. As you read through the autobiographical portion of this book, you will find that all these forces are at work when there are details or timelines missing. Perhaps you will relate.

Although much of my story came back to me over the course of healing, much of it hasn't. I have learned to be OK with this, and at times—even grateful.

Throughout my journey of healing, I have had to reconcile what I thought to be true with what I have been told by family members who, at long last, saw fit to give me details about my life that helped me dismantle the falsehoods in my story. Other times, I assembled the pieces of my own memories and experiences combined with what I know to be true from

a psychological perspective. This is what I had to do in order to make sense of my own story—gaps be damned. It just might be what you have to do to make sense of your own story, too.

In some parts of the story, the parts from before I was born, we will immerse ourselves in the scenes as though we were a fly on the wall. I have constructed these stories and resulting emotions and behaviors of those involved by combining the accounts of the people closest to the events, as well as my training as a therapist. In using this technique, I hope to help you experience and understand the impact of the events and of their consequences.

In other areas, we will explore accounts offered from family with whom I became acquainted later in life. Admittedly, balancing their input with what I know to be true has been challenging. In some cases, it caused me tremendous pain as I came to grips with the disparity between what I thought was true and what *actually* happened.

I had spent a lot of time dismantling the dysfunction of my past, in addition to working through the lies I was told throughout my childhood. It was a heavy blow to have more lies revealed, and then work through their implications.

Perhaps you grew up in an atmosphere like I did, where family members lied and hid the truth from you. I was often told that what I experienced, saw or heard wasn't what I *actually* experienced, saw and heard. Consequently, I felt crazy for calling things out. Sometimes, I was even punished for it. It was isolating and very confusing. If that was your experience too, let me say, I am sorry that happened to you. And you are *not* crazy. I hope reading this book helps you feel validated and affirmed.

Despite all the things that "I know that I know," there are other places where I must leave gaps in the story. Even though healing has taken

place in my life, there are still missing pieces in my story and in the timeline. I have come to terms with this and have peace about it, although that has not always been the case.

As I mentioned earlier, it's normal to have such gaps when one's life is marked by chaos, trauma, abuse or neglect. Still other gaps are caused by my own successful attempts to numb and disconnect by using less-than-legal substances. (I am pretty sure I was drunk, high or maybe both my entire high school career). I'm not bragging nor making light of this—I'm simply calling into light that in my attempts to protect myself emotionally and get what I thought I needed, there were many times when I was my own worst enemy. There were times when I hurt others out of my own pain—which makes sense. Hurt people hurt people. But free people? Well, guess what they can do? They point others to the places where freedom can be found.

While sometimes story gaps can be frustrating, even unsettling, they often serve a real and necessary purpose. I think it is important to point out that our brains are created to protect us, and sometimes that means blocking our recall of certain situations or experiences. To my knowledge, there is not any research that states we must unearth *every* memory in order to find freedom and healing. It is important that I tell you this because you need to know that freedom and healing are possible, *even if you can't remember your entire story*. Know that sometimes, the gaps we encounter, as unsettling as they might be, could actually be gifts from God—little shelters of protection along the way. Sometimes the gaps are places where the information, were it to be exhumed, would hold nothing but heartache and disappointment, of little to no value in our healing, growing and learning. Trust that what needs to be revealed for your healing will make its way into the light.

HOW TO USE THIS BOOK

Because there are some detailed accounts of trauma in my story, I want to offer a word of caution. As you read through this, you may find some portions of the book triggering, meaning it reminds you of a portion of your story that causes deep pain or intense anxiety. I promise to do my best to warn you when we are about to wade into those dark waters.

Sprinkled throughout the book you will find a few questions, prompts and suggestions to help you engage with your own story. If at any time those become overwhelming, simply skip them or put the book down completely and come back when you feel you have the emotional margin to do so. But please keep a journal or notebook handy for anything you might want to jot down for later, or to answer some of the questions in the book. This is an important tool I hope you don't omit from your journey. You don't have to be a writer or even a "journaler." Just write down thoughts, ideas, bullet points or even drawings that help you keep track of whatever comes up for you as you are reading.

To help you broaden your perspective on events in your story and the story of your family, you will find some assessments in Part Nine to help you think about what circumstances you encountered in your past that could be impacting you more than you know in your present. Taking the time to work through these will prove valuable to you. In fact, one was created especially for this book with the help of more than 60 therapists!

When you come to those assessments, if you are reading through the material alone, I encourage you to seek out someone to share your findings with. Depending on what new revelations surface, adding the support of a clinically trained counselor might be beneficial as well.

Perhaps most importantly, I need you to remember that no matter what you unearth from the generations before you or within your own life, no

matter what revelations you discover, none of that will ultimately define you. None of it is an irreversible sentence to a life you do not want to live. *You* get to decide. *You* have a choice. Together with God, *your journey is yours to create*. *Yours* to craft. *Yours* to protect.

I am so glad we get to do this together! I am here. And I am cheering you on.

PART TWO

Generations Past: Patterns Set in Motion

> "It's how we make sense of our past that matters the most."
> **DAN SIEGEL, MD**

My mother gave me up for adoption.

Twice.

While I didn't find out about this until just a few years ago, the implications of such a devastating relational blow were evident throughout my life. I knew she had placed me for adoption *once,* but the second time? That tidbit of therapy-worthy information eluded me for the first four and a half decades of my life.

Fortunately for me, there had been plenty of therapy-worthy moments from my childhood to keep me busy and my therapists gainfully employed. Collectively, our efforts afforded me the unique opportunity to amass several tools to aid in my digestion of this new morsel of genealogical intel.

Admittedly, I am still working out some of the details. The initial, piercing pain has settled to an occasional, dull ache that typically only surfaces in moments when my vulnerability is high and my emotional margins are low.

But what I have been able to work out so far is this: *what happened to me when I was a child is more than the consequence of my biological mother's choices.* The two of us were sort of "set up" for this outcome by choices and behaviors that established *patterns of dysfunction* long before either of us were born.

Let me explain: in families, *what is left unrepaired tends to be repeated.* Like a quirky smile or a bejeweled heirloom, we hand down our wounds from generation to generation. Science calls it Transgenerational Epigenetic Inheritance. The Bible calls it a generational curse. But both teach us

the same lesson: *to help ensure a healthier outcome for the generations that follow us, we must heal from what has harmed us.*

We either pass on our healing, or we pass on our hurting. That's not just some meme-worthy phrase. It's the reality of what I know from experience, both the personal and professional kind. And while the task can, at times, feel insurmountable, the truth is this: *it is possible to break generational patterns and alter the course of our own lives and those of our families for generations to come.*

We either pass on our healing, or we pass on our hurting.

To move forward in our journey, we must start in what seems like an unlikely place and board a ship bound for freedom with the hope of a brighter future.

But before we go any further, take a moment and consider your intention for reading this book and what you hope to take away at the end. Find paper and pen and write it down. (Yes, *actual paper* and *pen*.) If your intention changes and grows during your time with me in these pages, that is perfectly fine! Just set an initial intention here and now. Feel free to take your time with this. I will wait. Please don't skip this step. It will be important to reflect on your intention periodically as you read these pages and at the end of our time together.

CHAPTER 2 Coming to America

Antonio boarded the steamship, Giulio Cesare, with nothing but a strong back, flimsy suitcase and the dream of building a future in the United States of America. The March on Rome was less than a year behind him along with a lost sense of autonomy and control, now that Mussolini was in power. Antonio might've been a simple laborer, but he saw the writing on the wall for his country. He knew that if any hope of a free and fruitful future was to be found, it wouldn't be in his beloved Italy.

As Antonio walked his stocky frame through the narrow bridge that temporarily connected the ship to dry land, his hopes for the future grew with each step. When his feet reached the ship's deck he realized that with those last two steps, he was officially the furthest from home he'd ever been in his 24 years of existence. And it felt...fine. *Si Sente Bene*.

As he stepped up to the very front of the ship, Antonio inhaled the sea air, felt the dampness on his face from the humidity of the hot July day and tasted the salty spray on his lips. He had no sooner closed his eyes to imagine what future was ahead of him when he felt the forceful jolt of departure. Pressing his body into the furthest tip of the deck, he looked

down and noticed the ripple of rings that expanded from the bow of the ship as its mass pulled away from shore, away from life as he knew it.

I'm sure it didn't occur to him that much like the ripple effect in the water, Antonio himself was a massive force, pressing into the future to set off a ripple effect for generations to come.

This was my great grandfather. And perhaps, if he had had his way, I would have never been born.

A WHOLE NEW WORLD

Antonio arrived in the United States after a long and crowded journey across the sea, nearly six weeks from the last time he stood solidly on dry land. It was said in the stories he told that Ellis Island looked like nothing he'd ever known. The sights, smells and sounds were intoxicating. Yet he had no interest in falling in love with New York. Antonio had a plan and that plan required him to find his way to the middle of this new country. He was headed to St. Louis, Missouri.

Antonio knew what he would require in order to make his dream a reality... First, a job. Then, a wife. Fortunately for Antonio, his brother Pietro and his friend Garrera had arrived in the United States nearly a year before him. They were both already established. It was Garrera who would connect Antonio with a place to stay; brother Pietro would help with employment and, consequently, an introduction to a rapidly growing Italian community with a plethora of good Italian girls from which to choose a wife. While many of the women were *molto bella* (very beautiful) by any man's standards, none of them drew Antonio's big brown eyes nor won his favor.

While finding a wife and having a family of his own would be a dream come true, first and foremost, Antonio need a place to live. When my

great-grandfather came to the United States, it was during a time when sponsorship was needed, meaning an immigrant needed someone already in the country who would be a sort of guarantor—someone to take responsibility for them, to vouch for them.

The happy consequence of the sponsorship requirement for Antonio was that it gave him a ready-made community of other Italians as well as family, providing a rapid sense of belonging amidst the expectations, chaos and stress of acculturation. In the Italian American community in St. Louis, it also was customary for established residents to take in newcomers as boarders.

Antonio was taken in by Angelo and Lucia and their two children, Albert and Julie. The couple had settled in St. Louis some time ahead of him. And so, it was through the "Italian grapevine" (pun intended) that Angelo and Lucia connected with Antonio. They had a room to rent and renting it to Antonio seemed like the logical thing to do. It benefited them financially and gave Antonio a roof over his head.

Things were working out for Antonio. He had a job and a good place to live. He was building relationships in the community, making friends, finding a church and weaving himself into the fabric of America as it wove itself into him. All that was missing was a family of his own. I can only imagine how much watching his host family with their children deepened his longing for a place his heart could truly call home.

ANGELO AND LUCIA

Lucia was a first generation born Italian American who was no stranger to the challenges of living in a new country. By today's terms, we would say her parents were essentially trafficked to America. They were sponsored with the promise of a future if they would help settle a town in Arkansas. But each breath they took seemed to have a price tag, a debt

to be paid to the company store which left them perpetually in debt to those who brought them to the U.S.A. That is, until a blessing came in the form of an Italian priest who realized what was really taking place was the oppression of many people, and he liberated them from Arkansas to Missouri.

In Missouri, Lucia found a new home and hope for her future. She fell in love, at a tender age, around 15 (though likely commonplace for that time in history) and planned to marry her love when he returned from the war. Sadly, that day never came. His life ended all too soon in battle. Lucia must have been devastated—her hopes and dream of the future passing with her love.

Perhaps it was financial hardship or merely a sign of the times, but Lucia's future was then decided upon by her parents who promised her to a man who himself had immigrated from Italy. A man named Angelo. She was seventeen. Angelo was thirty.

What devastation to the heart of a young girl. The sort of emotions Lucia must've been forced to bury along with her first love likely caused a pain from which anyone would struggle to recover.

This kind of sorrow and loss can get imbedded in your very soul, seeping into the fabric of who you are, *"Into the DNA"* as one might say. The climate of her family and the times themselves didn't afford the luxury of expressing such emotions for a girl of Lucia's means. With nowhere to go with such emotions, one does what one must do to function: shut off and shut down in order to move on with the new life that had been assigned her. Only a powerful force would be able to reach into her heart and breathe life into what felt dead. A power that for Lucia, Angelo sadly did not possess.

Nonetheless, Angelo and Lucia set about creating a life together. I don't know much about Angelo; save to say I think he was a good man, a good

provider, not unkind. Angelo was likely eager to make a life for himself in the United States. And for Angelo, having children was a big part of that. I would imagine Lucia felt the same. And it wasn't long before they welcomed their first child, a girl they named Julie. It would take a few years, but eventually they would welcome a son, Alberto, into their world.

RESTLESS HEARTS

It seemed as though Lucia had decided to fully commit to this new life with Angelo, even though she hadn't chosen it for herself. Her sorrow over love lost was buried but most likely was not forgotten.

Human nature would suggest that perhaps her heart had never fully followed suit. Whatever laid dormant or suppressed would eventually demand to be expressed. The deeper emotions always do, whether we want them to or not.

As time went by, Antonio must have noticed the restlessness in Lucia. Perhaps he found it similar to his own, the desire for more, the hope of something bigger. And it drew him in. Whatever those conversations were like, sharing of heartache, feeling homesick or restlessness, they were the kind of conversations that built intimacy.

When a person feels unseen or unheard for a long time, it's inevitable that the one who finally helps them feel known becomes important. It is the truest act of intimacy to help someone feel fully known and fully loved. I think Lucia believed that's what Antonio did for her. And whether Angelo was incapable of this or whether Lucia simply never gave him the opportunity to try, that deeper level of intimacy happened with Antonio.

I have often imagined those conversations; Antonio listening as Lucia told him of the arranged marriage, her heartbreak from what seemed a lifetime ago and believing her ability to be loved deeply, and to deeply love, died with that man on the battlefield.

Or Antonio's stories of how he missed home but felt he had no choice; either leave Italy or abandon hope of the free life he always dreamed of. He must've shared his longing for true love and a family of his own.

These are the places where vulnerabilities and desires meet, where the unaddressed brokenness can come face to face with compassion and understanding. It would seem that this was where Lucia's buried passions were exhumed.

Unfortunately, this is also where memories of family become fuzzy, (or so they say) and details become harder to find than a needle in a haystack. But knowing a thing or two about brokenness and having at least some of the pieces to put together from family, here's the picture I see.

Lucia, while committed to Angelo and her family in most senses of the word, never felt fully committed to her marriage at a heart and soul level. Feeling less alive after losing her true love, she left a difficult home life as a mere teenager for what was ultimately a different kind of tumultuous life with Angelo. Her grief over the death of the future she had dreamt of went unexpressed, but never unfelt.

Because memories are short, secrets are precious and stories are decades, even a century old, no one seems to have a clear idea how it all happened, except to say that Lucia eventually left Angelo for Antonio. OK, "left" is a mild word. The story goes they "ran away together" to Tennessee.

Initially, Lucia left her children with her sisters. It's hard to guess why she would leave them. Maybe as a single woman, with two children in 1927

with nothing but uncertainty and this new love to cling to, she would've had very little means to support them. Perhaps she felt no guarantees in her relationship with Antonio or where it would lead.

Then, there's the issue of religion. In Catholic families, things like divorce were frowned upon at best, and grounds for alienation at worst. But leaving your children? In the family's eyes (and likely society's) that was inexcusable. What a risk she took! I think I can understand why she did what she did, but I want to be clear that understanding and condoning are two different things. And I do not condone her decision. In fact, I grieve the ripple effect it set off, especially for her daughter, Julie. Such long reaching consequences. But regardless of Lucia's reasons or motives, her choice to leave her children with her sisters set off a pattern of parental abandonment that reached decades into the future of our family.

Lucia's history paints a picture of emotional trauma that created beliefs within her about herself and her outer world. Beliefs such as "People die and are to be forgotten." "I am more of something to be traded than a person to be treasured." "Emotions are a luxury I can't afford." While those are guesses on my part, her actions reveal I'm not far off.

Eventually, Antonio and Lucia returned, and Angelo granted Lucia a divorce. She took her children back from her sisters, too. But the bond of sisterhood was torn apart and never fully repaired; they would never forgive Lucia for abandoning her children to them. From then on, Lucia was basically without close family, outside of her two children and of course, Antonio.

I can only imagine what this felt like to Julie and Albert. Not only did they feel abandoned by their mother for a time, but from what I understand, they didn't really see their father after the divorce either. Today we know what impact fatherlessness can have on a child. The human condition isn't one that has changed really, not from a heart and mind

perspective anyway. Father wounds, like the ones Julie and Albert experienced, are the kind that cut deep. This is another generational pattern that reached on through to the generations that followed.

At the end of the day, I think Lucia believed she could correct her mistake by marrying Antonio. And, in 1928, that's exactly what she did. So, Lucia left Angelo and became Antonio's wife. Eventually, she became my great-grandmother.

A NEW FAMILY

With the ink freshly dried on the marriage license, and Lucia reunited with her children, the four of them began the tough journey to becoming a family. Sadly, Antonio struggled with becoming an instant father. It was as though he had vowed internally that while he would provide the necessities for Lucia's children, he would not be a father to them, not in the deeper ways one needs a father.

While Antonio's decision to maintain emotional distance from Lucia's children was an internal one, it inevitably leaked out into the open. While perhaps no explicit messages were ever given, the implicit — what's expressed through actions (or lack of actions)—often speaks loudest. Tone of voice, a look, a lack of engagement or acknowledgment would've been apparent to bright children like Julie and Albert, who no doubt desired a father figure.

No one knows for certain if Lucia really knew what was in Antonio's heart. But if she did know, she never showed it. Maybe she believed that given time, he would change his mind. Perhaps she believed that if she could just be a good enough wife and they could be good enough children, then Antonio would change his mind, or more importantly, change his heart.

Oh, how many chain reactions of devastation are ignited by unrealistic expectations and holding on to the hope that reality is something other than what it really is.

Despite all the changes and loss they experienced, Julie and Albert were young, vibrant children. Julie, the eldest at age ten and Albert only eight, were excited to be back with their mom and anxiously anticipated a relationship with their new stepfather. But it wasn't long before they were experiencing some of those external consequences from Antonio's internal decision to stay detached.

At the time, no one seemed to fully understand just how much of a necessity fatherly nurturing is to a child. Some in my family said that while Antonio never physically or verbally abused Julie and Albert, he remained cold and unattached. We now know the deeper implications of emotionally-distant parenting on children throughout their lifespan. This, coupled with the absence of a biological father, would be a toxic cocktail for any child's development. It proved toxic for Julie and Albert. It opened a channel for layers of dysfunction to grow and permeate for the generations to come.

What Julie and Albert experienced are the kind of ruptures in relationship that create false self-narratives. No matter how much our parents' choices aren't about us, we deeply internalize them. While our head may mature beyond those beliefs, it can be very difficult to get our inner child to catch up and believe the same thing.

Eventually, Julie and Albert would leave home. Julie married into alcoholism, which would set off a ripple effect for her own children. Albert joined the military. Apparently, he preferred to fight a literal battle in the Second World War over remaining in the battle at home. I guess it's easier to fight a war when you understand the rules of engagement and know who the real enemy is.

If you find it challenging to keep track of "who's who" in my family tree, you're not alone. Go to page 347 for a quick Generations/Family Relationships Chart for reference whenever you need help.

YOUR TURN: Reflect. Engage. Write.

OK, My New Friend, I'm anxious to continue the journey with you, but I'd like to take a slight pause and give you a chance to "talk" for a moment. This will be the first of many opportunities throughout this book for *you* to set pen to paper as you reflect on the questions presented. Please hear my loudest encouragement for you to engage whenever these opportunities arise. **What you write about your own story, as it's prompted by what you read in these pages, will result in some of your most powerful takeaways from our time together.**

While we won't *always* have opportunities set within the content of this book to ask questions and ponder the implications of the story as it may relate to your own, I do hope throughout your time reading, you will give yourself an opportunity to ask yourself questions and write down anything your reading stirs. (Maybe consider going through the book with a friend.)

I wish we could have a real conversation about what you've read up to this point. Here are the questions I would ask:

- What do you suspect could've helped Lucia as a teen experiencing love lost?
- Have you already begun to form some guesses about what choices and behaviors will have the farthest-reaching impact?
- What in the story can you already see as problematic?

- In what ways could Lucia's decisions set Julie and Albert up for problems later in life?
- Are you beginning to see the truth behind the saying "we're only as sick as our secrets?"
- What have you read up to this point that may cause you to wonder about circumstances in your own story?

Consider taking some time to record your answers—if not here, then in a journal.

If you need time to process, particularly if this is rubbing up against something in your own story, feel free to stop here and pick up the story when you're ready.

CHAPTER 3 Blood Is Thicker Than Water

While Lucia (now Lucy) worked diligently to make their new situation feel like a "normal" family, Antonio (now, Tony) desperately wanted a child of his own. Finally, in June of 1932, his prayers were answered, and they welcomed Maria (Marie) into their world.

There was all the anticipated joy of a new baby, but Marie's arrival also brought tremendous resentment and anger from Julie and Albert, though their resentment wasn't *really* about Marie. Sadly, it would all become directed at her.

As I've listened to the stories about Marie and her siblings, it seemed that no matter how much Marie tried, she never felt like she fit in with her siblings. Lucy and Tony over-compensated to make up for it. They gave Marie favored status in Julie and Albert's eyes, which, in my understanding, backfired and further incited her siblings' disdain for her. As I listened to the stories about Marie's behavior, it also seemed that Lucy and Tony may have contributed to some of Marie's more bratty behaviors, as well.

For all the times Tony treated Julie and Albert as the ones who didn't belong, they learned well how to pass that on to Marie. And it settled deep within her. A little girl never quite accepted or approved of by those she so desperately wants approval from will eventually grow into a young lady who struggles to accept herself or know where she fits in this life. This is what I would call an identity wound—a blow that strikes at the very core of who you believe you are.

Eventually, all the confusion, restlessness and rejection helped her write her own unhealthy and false self-narrative. In time, that searching and uncertain little girl would grow to become a woman who struggled deeply. Always searching. Always uncertain.

Marie became the rebel, the troublemaker. I'm not sure at what age it happened, but my guess is that at some point Marie made an internal agreement with herself about what she could and couldn't get from her family. Not an agreement that was conscious. Rather, one that whispered to her unconscious mind. One that might sound like this: "I'm not wanted here, so, I will find somewhere that I am."

From then on, Marie pursued affirmation and acceptance with a passion and hunger that could not be deterred. She was out of control. Eventually, at 14, she thought she had found what she longed for: a sense of belonging and feeling loved that was so strong she was willing to carry out the ultimate act of rebellion to make sure it was hers to keep.

MARIE (AND CHARLIE)

One thing Marie had going for her (or perhaps against) was her external beauty and charm. From childhood, her beauty was remarked upon by family, friends and strangers alike. With her big, hazel-green eyes and thick, wavy auburn hair and olive skin, she was a striking presence in the room. And despite her insecurities, she carried herself with confidence

and a defiant sort of happiness, as though she refused to admit to the world, and possibly to herself, the pain she carried.

She also looked much older than her 14 years, and consequently blended in with the older crowd. Perhaps they filled the void her siblings left in her life. In any case, hanging out with the cool cats and kittens opened the door for her to catch the eye of a very handsome, very charismatic upper classman named Charles, or "Charlie." Charlie stood out in a crowd. Taller than most of the boys his age and broad shouldered, with bright blue eyes and dark blonde hair, it would've been difficult for Marie not to notice him, too. He was just the right combination of good looks, charm and bad boy demeanor to draw Marie's attention, and perhaps to appeal to her rebellious side.

I don't know much about Charlie, but I know Marie loved him. I think he loved her, too. I believe if he had his way, they would've stayed together. I also believe the attention he gave her may have just saved her life in that space and time.

It didn't take long for Marie to make Charlie the center of her world, with no concern for the fact that she was only 14 and he was 18.

She must've known her parents would never accept the relationship, but to end it would have likely felt like death to her. He was breathing life and love into her—a powerful force that she would want to protect at all costs. Marie seemed to be taking a page from her mother's book, choosing the relationship that she felt she needed over what was best. She didn't realize that she was reenacting the same destructive choices her mother, Lucy, had made; engaging in a relationship that would cause so much damage to the people she loved and damage herself in the process, as well.

Instead, Marie gave in to the part of herself that couldn't let Charlie go. At 14, she stole her sister Julie's identification. Armed with illegitimate "proof" that she was of legal, consenting age, and looking like

a young lady much older than her actual years, Marie and Charlie ran away to get married. Guess where they ran to? That's right. Tennessee. (Talk about your generational patterns! Remember, this is exactly where Lucy and Tony went when they ran.)

I'm certain these two high schoolers had no idea what they would do next or where they would go, once they were husband and wife. I wonder if they had fantasies about what their married life would look like or how they would make their way in the world. Although, being in love like they were, I can't imagine they cared.

But their plan was not the plan Tony and Lucy had for their little girl. Eventually, the young lovers were found and brought back home. Despite all their protests and professions of deep love for one another, Tony and Lucy had the marriage annulled.

I think what surprised me the most when I learned this story was Lucy's seemingly cold, dismissive response to Marie. She had buried her own heartbreak over her first, lost love so far down that she was unable to recognize the heartbreak and need in her own daughter.

YOUR TURN: Reflect. Engage. Write.

Dear Friend, when those you love experience grief or pain, whether self-inflicted or from someone else, and if that experience reminds you of something similar you went through, reach down deep and connect with what that was like for you. Then, respond to your loved one from that place. But remember! We can only do this well if we have healed from that pain. That is when we're most effective.

If you can recall an experience like that, spend a few moments writing about it now.

A BOND NOT EASILY BROKEN

Once they were brought back home, even though the marriage was over, it took a lot of work to keep Marie and Charlie from one another. I'm unsure of the circumstances surrounding this, or how long they were gone. But I do know that it wasn't long after they returned that Marie told her parents she was pregnant. The timing of her pregnancy remains a mystery. Did they run away to marry because she was pregnant? Did she get pregnant while they were away? Did she get pregnant after they were forced to come home and their marriage was annulled? Those questions will forever remain unanswered. But I have my suspicions, and my suspicion is that she was already pregnant when they ran away, another generational pattern that repeated in my family. As for the baby she gave birth to nine months later, that was my mother, Cathy.

It's hard not to think about the begging and pleading Marie (my grandmother) must've done with her parents to let her and Charlie stay married. It is one thing to be denied access to your love, another thing completely when you're literally carrying a piece of him inside you. So many questions have flooded my mind over the years. What could have possibly motivated my great-grandparents to keep my grandparents apart? Was it possible they had no idea of the damage it would cause?

In an Italian Catholic family and community, wouldn't it have been more acceptable to allow them to stay together and try to make a go of it? Wouldn't my great-grandparents' energies have been better spent on trying to help Marie and Charlie learn how to be a family with their new baby in tow?

Since anger and control issues are both a legacy in my family, I can't help but wonder if pure, unadulterated rage over her blatant disregard for their rules wasn't part of the motivation behind keeping them apart. I think they were attempting to dole out consequences for a disobedient child. In reality, she abandoned her childhood when she ran away and

married Charlie, and got pregnant, or perhaps ran away to marry him *because* she was already pregnant. Regardless of what order those things occurred, the consequences were already there, naturally occurring.

A MISSING PIECE

To this day, I want to believe with everything in me that I'm missing what would help me see Tony's and Lucy's choices in a different light. Perhaps if I had some additional information, I would be able to see why they acted the way they did. I want to believe they had no idea just how far reaching their decisions would go in perpetuating a cycle of dysfunction in the family.

But throughout my exploration of the stories within my own family, I see that time and time again emotional intelligence, and by default, empathy and an ability to connect deeply, were critical missing pieces. It was the thing that everyone needed and wanted so desperately. But they couldn't name what they didn't know.

In today's world, we know the importance of emotional intelligence (EQ). In fact, study after study tells us that the greatest indicator of success, not only in relationships but in business and nearly every other aspect of life, is most often determined by our EQ rather than our IQ. Emotional intelligence wasn't even a definable or quantifiable thing back in those days. I'm sure that in those days, many families possessed it intrinsically, and as such were able to naturally pass it along to their children and consequently, their children's children.

However, EQ wasn't something that was called out or recognized for the significance and powerful impact it possessed. I don't think it came up in mainstream conversation like it does today. And it most certainly wasn't a focus of "personal growth." I'm not sure there was much intentional talk about "personal growth" in any form. Likely, it was more of

an unnameable luxury when times were hard and priorities were more tangible.

From my great-grandmother to my grandmother, to my mother and then on to me, it would seem that with each generation, there was a steady decline in value of self and an unhealthy perspective of worth which made way for a deep darkness to creep in through so many avenues: drugs, alcohol, toxic relationships, complete lack of self-care, a view of a God who couldn't possibly be accepting or loving—and certainly not trustworthy.

Perhaps because it was all so familiar from one generation to the next, those toxic behaviors were viewed as normal rather than the destructive forces they truly were. As a result, pain and shame were normalized too, which ultimately ruled out the possibility that one generation to the next could offer empathy—the thing that might have made it possible for people to heal and change under the umbrella of grace. Sadly, no healing happened.

CHAPTER 4 Patterns Continue into Modern Times

MARIE AND CATHY

When my mother (Cathy) was born, my grandmother (Marie) was 15. *Fifteen*.

I'm not sure about you, but I know a few 15-year-olds, many who aren't even equipped to babysit, let alone equipped to be mothers. (If we had room, we could go into the science of how under-developed our brains are at that age; ill-equipped to make the "big" decisions.)

After Marie had Cathy, life became more and more distressing for everyone in the home. Here's what I'm told: Marie desperately wanted to figure out a way to have a relationship with Charlie, but that was not to be. Tony and Lucy were incredibly intrusive in Marie's attempts to be a mother and made it all too easy for her to shirk her responsibilities. With Charlie absent, Tony and Lucy felt an unspoken guilt over Cathy being raised without a father. (Cue irony.) So, they over-compensated, spoiling her and smothering her. Sound familiar?

Tony and Lucy often lamented to family about the strife Marie had brought to their home and to the family. The tension was palpable and relentless. From the stories I've been told, it would seem that Tony and Lucy couldn't let it go. The stories told paint a picture of them withholding their affection from Marie and redirecting it toward Cathy. This set off yet another covert pattern of behavior in the family. As I type this I can once again recall when I was little and would get in trouble, or when the adults in my home were upset with one another, people would withhold affection from each other as punishment, instead, directing their love toward someone else in the family. It was one of the most anxiety-producing elements of my childhood, at times lasting for days, sometimes weeks.

The heartbreaking part of this is that, for all of us, when we make a mistake, what prevents us from feeling like we are the mistake is the ability of our caregivers to continue to show us love—even when they are angry and upset. But when the punishment for the mistake involves emotional deprivation, with no repair, there is far more harm done than good. Our identity takes a hit, and shame takes root. This was true for Marie.

With the strain between Marie and her parents, she grew resentful of her own daughter for seemingly taking her place and resentful of her parents for destroying her relationship with Charlie. She may have even been resentful of Charlie for not fighting harder. But my guess is that she resented herself the most.

It's important to mention yet another pattern repeating itself here: Fatherlessness. Julie and Albert basically grew up without their father and without the attention of a stepfather once Tony had his own child to focus on. Marie lost Tony's attention when she gave birth to Cathy. And Cathy's father, Charlie, would be absent for much of her life.

Resentment was a legacy, too. In so much as Marie's siblings resented her, she resented Lucy and Tony for denying her a future with her love, Charlie. Although they were mother and daughter, not sisters, Tony and

Lucy treated Marie and Cathy as siblings and because of this Marie not only resented them, but eventually turned her resentment toward her own daughter, feeling as though she had taken her place in their hearts. As Cathy grew, Marie infected her with resentment and disdain for Tony and Lucy, as well.

With each passing year, the evidence of Cathy's resentment was vocalized and obvious in her rebellion. Consequently, the tensions in the home grew as well. Marie's half-brother Albert, back from the Navy and married with a child of his own, had moved into the adjoining duplex, close to home yet slightly removed from all the chaos. But walls were thin and voices were loud, so Albert would often hear the fighting next door and, as the story goes, eventually felt compelled to intervene.

During one particularly cacophonous encounter, Albert set out to put an end to the confrontations for good. Here is what I know of the events of that evening:

"What is all the screaming about over here?!" Albert boomed as he burst through his parents' front door.

He was surprised to see not only Marie posed to verbally pounce on Lucy, but Cathy standing at her side equally ready for battle.

His surprise entrance knocked everyone off their game for a moment, but Marie quickly recovered. "This is none of your business, brother," Marie hissed. The familial reference dripped with disdain. "Go back to your side," she concluded before turning her back on him to face Lucy.

"I'm not going anywhere until this is settled respectfully. She is my mother, too," he said, pointing to Lucy. "And I'm sick and tired of hearing you talk to her like this. Do you realize the bad example you're setting for Cathy?" (Pointing to my mother) "How do you expect her to treat you any differently than she sees you treating your own mother?"

(Exactly, Albert. Exactly.)

But Cathy had already begun lashing out at Marie. As I said before, they interacted more often as siblings than parent-child. Albert's interventions were too-little-too-late, which should've come as no surprise to him since he had little in the way of solid relationships to stand on with Marie or Cathy.

With each passing year, and particularly with the onset of teenage angst, Cathy's frustrations and restlessness with her home life deepened. It was just as Cathy was entering those years that Marie left her with Lucy and Tony. In part, I can see why Marie eventually gave up attempts at parenting. Lucy and Tony never really gave Marie a chance to be a parent.

When Marie left, it was for a man named Roger. Later, a relative told me that Marie had said, "I feel like this is my last shot at being happy."

But "happy" is an illusion when you're not sure of who you are or your true worth. While Marie said she was searching for "happy," I think what she was really searching for was wholeness.

Happiness or wholeness, whatever her motivations were, Marie married Roger. Based on my knowledge of the situation, I believe she married not for love or money or security, but because Roger worshiped the ground she walked on. Roger's willingness to put her on a pedestal and offer constant affirmations likely helped with her unmet need for acceptance and love. Perhaps she hoped the way Roger saw her could eventually become the way she saw herself.

But by that time, all the relational chaos she had already experienced in her life had caused Marie to establish a pattern of escape through alcohol and prescription drugs, even before she met Roger.

What started as a lack of connection, peace and safety in Marie's external environment eventually grew into shame and internal uncertainty about her identity and worth. Drugs and alcohol became her way to cope, and to numb from the pain she carried. Sadly, her relationship with Roger didn't help. Oddly, it seemed to have the opposite effect. Maybe she felt that she could never be the person he thought she was. In any case, my grandmother's addiction was the beginning of patterns of addiction in our family for years to come.

Alcohol and prescription drugs were the end of Marie. As often occurs with long-term substance abuse, Marie developed a physiological need for drugs and alcohol beyond her mental and emotional need for them. Eventually, they consumed her.

Later I would learn that Marie suffered from anxiety and depression as well, though there wasn't much done about it back then. And all of what she struggled with has been passed from generation to generation. Looking back at what my great-grandmother Lucy endured in her own life, I can see the seeds of depression in her story as well.

That's why I believe it's important to know our stories, to know what contributes to our beliefs about ourselves, others, our world and even God.

It is important to know what our inherited vulnerabilities are so we can design a life that minimizes the risk of repeating unhealthy and unhelpful behaviors and habits. Knowledge combined with action creates change. We can change things for ourselves and for the generations that follow us if we're willing to be honest with ourselves and to do the good, hard work of healing.

Generations/Family Relationships Chart reference, page 347

YOUR TURN: Reflect. Engage. Write.

My Dear Friend, it's your turn again. Here are a few more questions to ponder. Remember, to get the most out of these sections of the book, you will want to write your answers in your journal. You might want to come back to them later!

- What additional patterns/concepts stuck out to you from this portion of the story?
- What do you know about the generations who have gone before you?
- Are there things you struggle with in your present life that are a mystery to you because you can't seem to connect them to anything you've personally experienced? If so, perhaps some investigation into the generations before you can shed some light on where the struggle really began, and who it began with. Research shows there is a genetic component to things like mental illness, addiction, and from what I've studied and experienced, even trauma and shame.
- After reading this far, are there things you suspect you have unintentionally passed on to your kids? Or if you do not have children, are there things you are beginning to recognize that have been passed on to you?

If so, please don't feel hopeless about it. You can help them while you are helping yourself. Sometimes that requires getting professional help too. A willingness to get help is a sign of successful and healthful decision making!

CHAPTER 5 Pattern Turns Deadly

MARIE'S GOODBYE

Marie's substance abuse problem grew bigger than she could handle and eventually, it took her life. It has been said that Marie wrote a note to Roger telling him that she was sorry and that he deserved better. A final declaration of what she really believed about herself. With the note written and Cathy in the hands of Tony and Lucy (conveniently on their way out of the country to visit Tony's hometown in Italy), it is difficult to look to see Marie's death as anything other than suicide, even though that word has intentionally never been spoken by the family.

Although Marie might have hoped the physical distance would spare Cathy from pain, the reality was that no distance could protect Cathy from this tragedy. When Tony, Lucy and Cathy arrived in New York anticipating to board the ship that would take them to Italy, word was waiting that there had been a tragic "accident" back home. They immediately boarded a flight back to St. Louis and back to a whole new reality for all of them.

I believe that for Cathy, Marie's death was the ultimate in abandonment. While Marie had been emotionally absent in Cathy's childhood and adolescence, she was now wholly and fully absent.

I wish Marie had been able to make the connection between all that she missed emotionally and relationally growing up and the pain she felt as an adult. I wish there had been someone to help her see it. And I wish that her parents had come clean with their own mistakes and helped Marie find healing. With the help and honesty of her parents and her own honesty, she might have found the keys to unlock the chains of misery she walked in on a daily basis. It would have been a privilege to share that Marie was able to repair and renew her connection with Cathy, which would prevent further wounds for the generations to come in my family.

FINDING CHARLIE

Somehow, during all the chaos and pain, Cathy reached out and contacted her father, Charlie. Unbeknownst to Lucy and Tony, Cathy made arrangements to be near her father and her siblings (Charlie had remarried and now had other children.) Lucy and Tony were frustrated by what must've been seen by them as an act of deception, but they were already struggling with Cathy's constant rebellion and, with the added stress of losing their daughter, they had no energy to protest.

Shockingly, Charlie came to Marie's funeral to be with Cathy. And I must give him credit for that. As unwanted as his attendance was and how undoubtedly awkward it must have made things for everyone (except Cathy), he chose to be there for his daughter and to pay respects to his first love, his first wife.

It's unclear if Charlie and Marie kept in touch much, but I tend to think they did in some fashion. Perhaps Marie even encouraged Cathy to

connect with Charlie and her siblings from time to time. After all, this would make sense. Marie knew all too well the ache of wanting to connect with siblings yet being unable to. Perhaps this was her way of trying to spare Cathy some of the pain she had felt.

Cathy was 16 when Marie died. With her mother gone and little desire to stay with Lucy and Tony, a new question surfaced for Cathy. "Would it be possible for me to be part of a real family? With a dad and a mom and siblings?" Oh, how much she wanted this to happen. It was the cry of her heart for years. With Charlie remarried and siblings in the picture, the family she hoped for must have seemed possible.

I wonder if she felt the need to change or reinvent herself to fit in, to earn their love. I wonder if she felt the tension from her siblings as she attempted to interject herself into a family that was relatively foreign to her and she to them. I wonder if she felt the resentment from her stepmother (that would become apparent later) from the start. Admittedly, those questions stem from my own experiences at points in my own story.

Sadly, attempts to live with her father and stepmother didn't last very long. I can't say for sure what the tensions were, but I can guess.

In fact, I experienced something very similar. Just like in my story, it didn't work out for Cathy and eventually she went back to live with her grandparents ... and, then back to live with her father and stepmother. And on and on, bouncing from place to place when conflicts were too intense, never really feeling like she belonged, like she was home.

CATHY

Having experienced it in my own life, I can almost feel the frenetic pace at which Cathy searched for that deeper sense of belonging. The less she was able to find it with family, the more she rebelled and acted out. It

isn't surprising to me to hear stories about my mother being "wild" or a "partier." Like her own mother, the emotional needs that went unmet eventually became too much. So, she numbed them with alcohol and unhealthy choices. Her behaviors were understandable, because eventually, when you can't find what your soul so desperately needs in a healthy way, you'll settle for a cheap substitute. But it's an illusion, like relying on saltwater to quench your thirst in the moment, while the truth is it will leave you thirstier than before.

The deeper Cathy's wounds grew, the wilder her behaviors grew, too. Consequently, that became the way her family saw her: Wild.

I realize that leaves a lot to the imagination. So, let's just say, that most of what you might imagine when you hear the word "wild" was probably accurate: promiscuity, alcohol abuse, lies and deception. There weren't many boundaries she wasn't willing to cross.

I'm certain her reasons for being wild were deeper than mere disobedience and willfulness. Chaos can become a way of life, a place of familiarity and comfort. For Cathy, I think this was the case. In a bizarre way, I think the chaos of that wild life felt safe for Cathy. At the very least, familiar, something she knew how to navigate. She had learned to find function in the dysfunction of her homelife as a child so even if there had been stability with her dad and stepmom, it would have felt foreign and unsafe. After all, you only trust what you know, even if all you know is unhealthy.

Can you imagine the toxic level of shame Cathy carried on a daily basis? Imagine what it might have been like in the early 1950s to be a girl raised without a father. I would guess that whether implicitly or explicitly, she was constantly faced with reminders that she was "different" and didn't quite fit in. After a while, not fitting in becomes your identity. Everything you do is rooted in the belief that you are different in the most broken sense of the word.

In her late teens, Cathy found her cheap alternative for connection through sexual relationships and what one might call "serial dating." Eventually, the ripple effect of her self-destructive behaviors and beliefs about herself would reach beyond Cathy and into my life. In fact, that frenetic search for connection is how I came into being.

YOUR TURN: Reflect. Engage. Write.

Dear Friend, it is here where we should pause and discuss something important. First, it is important to recognize that not all patterns handed down from one generation to the next are behavioral in nature. And, it isn't always situational dynamics that repeat themselves either. Often, it is a **belief** that repeats itself. It could be a *belief* about ourselves, others, the world and even God. Patterns of beliefs can be far more insidious and much more difficult to unearth than overt patterns of behaviors. While there is a sort of symbiotic relationship between the beliefs and behaviors, the beliefs we carry about ourselves tend to stay hidden within our internal environment.

Take, if you will, the example of my great-grandmother. Losing a deep love at such a tender age without so much as an acknowledgment of what happened can be life-altering. I believe it was for Lucy. It would be easy to come out of a situation like hers believing that what really mattered were family responsibilities and societal norms, not her feelings or the pain she was experiencing. A loss like that is a *trauma*. Unaddressed traumas have far-reaching implications. It would be a natural consequence for Lucy (Lucia) to see herself as merely a girl to be "married off." It would be difficult to develop a sense of empathy when you hadn't seen it modeled.

So, when the time came that Marie needed empathy, Lucy couldn't provide it. In the emotional economy of the family it was a "fend for yourself" environment, which Marie did. Then, the lack of empathy

and support Marie experienced from Lucy was passed on to Cathy, along with the legacy of bad choices and a belief that she wasn't worth the emotional investment. Lucy, Marie and Cathy never realized that a person can't give what they don't have.

Now, here are a few questions for you to consider.

- Are there things you've read up to this point that are making you curious about some things in your own story and the story of your family?
- What personal experiences are my story calling to mind?
- What, if anything, in your story are you seeing in perhaps a different light as you read this book?
- Is this story shining a light on any patterns in your own family?

Take a moment to write your answers down so you can reflect on them later.

PART THREE

In My Life: Patterns and Pain Repeating

CHAPTER 6 My Birth and Adoption Story

THE ORIGINAL VERSION OF THE STORY

My biological mom, Cathy, once told me that although she was terrified about having a baby, a part of her was happy as well. Despite the less-than-ideal-circumstances, she held some hope and joy for the life growing inside her, for me. Knowing the news of her pregnancy would not be well-received, she strategically waited a very long time to tell her grandparents. In her own words, "Practically until it was unavoidable." I can understand why she waited. Perhaps she didn't want the same fate as that of her own mother, fearful she would not get to parent her own child.

It was just into her sixth month of pregnancy, and with great trepidation, when Cathy finally came clean with her grandparents about her "condition." And in the blink of an eye, all her reasons for delaying the conversation became a reality. As the story she told me goes, straight out of the gate, they told her it would be best for everyone if she had an abortion. An abortion! It wasn't even legal in 1968. And in a Catholic

family, nonetheless! But, when they found out how far along she was, they quickly changed their tune and began pressuring her into adoption.

Cathy had no intention of agreeing to any of their suggestions. According to Cathy, the pressure was relentless, and they even went so far as to try and bribe her by offering to buy her a car and set her up in Chicago where she had previously wanted to go to nursing school. Finally, when she was eight months pregnant, they realized there was no convincing her that their way was best. So they kicked her out.

With little money or possessions to her name, Cathy took two jobs and worked them both practically up until the day she was ready to deliver. When the time came for her to give birth, she was admitted to a special home/hospital for unwed mothers, most of them teens.

Upon her release (our release), she went back to work after just a few days of recovery. Having no additional funds for childcare, Cathy recruited the help of her cousin Judy and Judy's husband, Ernie, to babysit me while she worked. (To help you keep everyone's familial role straight, Judy was the daughter of Julie, my grandmother Marie's sister.)

Judy and Ernie welcomed the distraction of a baby into their home. Unable to have children of their own and struggling through marital problems (in part, because of it) they happily turned all their focus to me. The lightheartedness of a baby was a welcome reprieve from their daily relational challenges. I would like to think that I was quite the delight!

With the prompting and encouragement of my great-grandparents, their energies quickly turned to how they could convince Cathy to let them adopt me. I think this was the first thing they had agreed on in a long time.

To help them build their case for adoption, on several nights when Cathy would get home from work at around two in the morning, Judy and Ernie would often convince her to let me stay and sleep rather than taking me out in the middle of the night. Feeling guilty, she would normally acquiesce.

I think the guilt and shame over leaving me with her cousins all those nights exacerbated her drinking and running wild; looking to numb her pain, or perhaps fill some hole in her soul. Maybe it was a little bit of both. And let's not gloss over the stress she must've been carrying as a new, single parent in 1968. All of the shame and distress led to a hopelessness that was too much for Cathy. The walls of the little home she tried to build for us were caving in. And no one was offering to help her hold them up, let alone repair them.

Eventually, life overwhelmed Cathy. When I was six months old, the stress, depression and anxiety that, for her, came with being a single mom, was more than she could handle. With little in the way of options and no longer able to handle the crushing weight of motherhood and the guilt and shame she carried, Cathy finally agreed to allow Judy and Ernie to adopt me. It's been said that they were initially excited to have a child, in part because they hoped becoming parents would breathe life into their marriage. Putting the responsibility to repair their marriage on an eight-pound-fourteen-ounce baby was unrealistic. They needed adult solutions for their adult problems.

Having divorced and then remarried in the hopes of having a better relationship, particularly with a child in the mix, Judy and Ernie's marriage was tense at best. Between Judy's volatile temper and the two of them constantly uncertain of what Cathy was going to do, I don't think settling into a "normal" family life (whatever that means) ever happened.

The turmoil intensified when Cathy reneged on the adoption and took me back– only to change her mind again and give me up a second time.

I can't imagine the emotional roller coaster this was for everyone in the family.

Still, Judy and Ernie gave it what they believed was their best shot at being good parents. Unfortunately, *we are limited in our ability to parent by the amount of healing we're able to do before we actually become parents. And Judy and Ernie each carried their own wounds and unaddressed dysfunctions. Eventually, all the stressors added up to divorce, and when I was five, they separated for good.*

ADOPTED—TWICE

It's sad that I never knew about Cathy reneging on my adoption, only to give me back to Judy and Ernie. It took 46 years for that piece of my story to reveal itself. Had I known sooner, it might have made my journey to healing less muddy. That information would've been incredibly beneficial in therapy as I worked to understand the root of some of my own struggles, particularly as it pertains to something called Attachment and Attachment Wounds, and the implication those wounds hold for virtually every relationship in our lives. In short, Attachment is how we learn to be secure about our relationships and Attachment Wounds are a type of trauma that occurs when parents (or caregivers) fail to adequately meet our needs. Examples include, but are not necessarily limited to, parent(s) being neglectful, rejecting, invalidating, unsupportive or emotionally unavailable. Healing these wounds is key in order to form healthy and fulfilling relationships as adults. In Parts Eight and Nine of this book, we will explore in depth what helps us heal.

For as much as they couldn't get it right in marriage, Ernie and Judy couldn't get it right in divorce either. Their split was far from amicable. It was downright hostile. Their inability to get along was a challenge for everyone, including my adopted grandmother, Julie (Judy's mom) and my adopted uncle, Corky (Judy's brother). Judy and I moved in

with them after the divorce. (Side note: if you're paying attention to the twisted, knotty branches of this family tree, you'll recognize that my "Grandma Julie" was really my "Great-Aunt Julie," Marie's older sister, making Cathy and Judy cousins.)

To Ernie's credit, I don't really remember him ever saying anything bad about Judy. His heavy sighs and facial expressions communicated a cascade of emotions as she would go on one of her tirades, which was quite often. Sometimes he would have stern words for her, typically to combat her venom, but always in a respectful way. But regardless of who was on the attack and who was on the defense, their most powerful weapon against one another was me.

As far as custody goes, it didn't look much different than all the traditional splits in those days. Every other weekend was spent with Ernie, with the occasional visit during the week for vacations and special occasions. There were phone calls when something important happened (or when I was in trouble) and a week of vacation together in the summer.

I often wished I could spend more time with Ernie to get away from the chaos in our new home. At first, it was wonderful! As a precocious six year old, I really enjoyed having the extra attention from my Grandmother Julie and Uncle Corky, as well as all the changes in our routine. But the newness soon wore off for everyone and tensions ran high once again when my grandmother (Julie) attempted to parent me over my mother (Judy).

Sound familiar?

By the time I was nine, there had been a steady decline in Judy's mental and even physical state. As a child, I wasn't sure why. I felt more and more the need to care for her. I was torn between wanting to be with Ernie more and feeling obligated to be with Judy, fearful that if I were not there, something horrible and irreversible would happen.

Sometimes, I refused to see Ernie even when I really wanted to because I felt like he didn't want me around. Perhaps that was because of things Judy said. Honestly, he really had no idea how to be a father to a daughter, or to anyone for that matter. The older I got, the less he knew what to do with me, which in my young head made sense because I had no idea what to do with myself, either.

UNSURE OF MY PLACE

With most everyone in our family working feverishly to keep all kinds of secrets from me (and some from themselves), people acted incredibly odd around me. There seemed to always be this low hum of frustration and aggravation when I was around, but I could never figure out why. Being a kid, I never assumed it was because of their own inner battles. I mistakenly assumed that since it seemed directed at me, it must've been my fault. Consequently, for most of my childhood, I walked around thinking I had done something wrong. I just couldn't figure out what it was. Of course, I hadn't done anything wrong.

The reality was that most of what I experienced with Judy was likely due to an undiagnosed disorder called Borderline Personality Disorder (BPD). People with borderline personality disorder often exhibit intense episodes of anger, depression, and anxiety. They have unpredictable moods and behaviors and tremendous difficulties in their relationships. The traits (or symptoms) of BPD occur on a sort of continuum—from those who exhibit severe and chronic traits, to those who might be better able to manage symptoms and function at a higher level. The idea of the possibility that Judy suffered from BPD was hinted at by a therapist I worked with briefly in my twenties as we talked through Judy's mood swings, manipulation, and at times, what seemed like outright cruel behavior toward me. The idea of BPD crystalized for me years later in graduate school when I became more familiar with the disorder.

In our new home, my Grandmother Julie and my Mom (Judy) shared a bedroom while Uncle Corky occupied the entire basement. Literally. I honestly can't ever remember going down there. Ever. Fortunately for me, this allowed me to have my own room, my place of escape.

Corky didn't work. I'm not sure why. I know he had been in Vietnam, but I don't know the real story of his life. I know he was an alcoholic with a volatile temper. Most of the time, I wasn't just his niece. I was his buddy too. Which for the most part was awesome, though not a "child-friendly" position to hold.

I was "the buddy" he took to the bowling alley with him. The buddy he let sit at the bar and sip his beers. The buddy he let pull the tabs off his lotto cards (and with whom he sometimes shared his winnings). The buddy he taught how to bowl and screamed at when I got it wrong or when he was too drunk and impatient to teach me the proper way to roll the ball. But he tried.

In an odd way, Uncle Corky and I were sort of kindred spirits. I think he sensed my struggle to feel as though I belonged in our family, and I think he related. Much like me, people didn't talk to him very often. They mostly talked about him. But rarely in his presence.

As I got older, I grew more certain that my family could not be trusted. Most of the time there was some level of tension in the air, but again I was pretty sure that was my fault since it seemed to always be present with family when I entered a room. Of course, now I know it wasn't because of me. It was because of the volume of secrets they were keeping, and the crushing weight many of them felt because of those secrets.

Regardless of the cost to me or to themselves, they were determined to keep each and every secret. Knowing some of those secrets now, I do believe many of my family members did what they did because they

were trying to protect me. Others were trying to protect each other. Some were trying to protect themselves.

Perhaps it was just as much about the way they kept the secrets as it was the secrets themselves. Outside of the context of nurturing relationships or providing a balance of really good things to counteract the really bad, I was left with no other alternative than to internalize all of the negativity, chaos and stress. Here's an example: as a young child, whenever I walked into a room where extended family was present, conversation would usually come to an abrupt halt. Or worse yet, they would continue speaking but switch to Italian and the only word I recognized was my name, said in conversations with scowls and tsking (You know, that "shaming sound" teachers and other adults make when they disapprove of something? Or someone?). Added to this was the confusion about exactly how I was related to them. In most families, you learn from a very young age who the cast of characters is in your family, and how you're all related. But in my family, those conversations didn't take place. There was simply an expectation that I would accept them as family and hold deep respect for them as such. At the time it felt very unsettling and added to my level of distrust for adults. In hindsight, I think they didn't know how to navigate the fact that my adoption had stayed in the family—they didn't want me to figure out that my cousin was actually my biological mother.

But...had they been able to smile in my direction, change the subject completely, or better yet, just focus on a connection with me when I walked into a room, it could have been different for me. Perhaps it would have emboldened me to trust, to feel cared for and accepted. Instead, their negative ways of relating to me deepened my attachment wounds.

Mostly, my bids for connection went unrecognized. In those moments of uncertainty, I worked to earn their positive regard. I can remember doing my very best to make them smile, laugh or soften, anything to feel

accepted, to feel "OK." I'd run and get pictures I drew, or papers with a teacher's red "A" at the top of the page. I would ask if I could get them something (a drink or snack) or if they wanted to play a game. I would give hugs and kisses. Sing songs. Perform dances I'd learned in my ballet and tap class. Anything my young mind could think of to change the direction of their conversation. But really, I was hoping to change their minds about me. I wanted to feel loved and like I fit in.

Generations/Family Relationships Chart reference, page 347

CHAPTER 7

Repair or Inherit

THE PROBLEMS WITH SECRETS AND SHAME

Everyone in my family was wrapped up in a strange sort of fear—they would just as soon talk about one another than to talk to one another. Mostly, they didn't want me to know the truth—about my adoption (two times)—and about the way they felt about Cathy and her choices. The list of secrets and side conversations included their disapproval for Judy and Ernie's divorce, the way both of my mothers were using alcohol and pills, for Julie, and how she was handling the behaviors of her adult children, or rather, wasn't handling it. All the turmoil, all the hushed whispers, the side-eyes, all of it was the result of ill-equipped people trying to understand what happened to our family. All. Of. The. Secrets. All of the shame.

Yet not a single soul thought to intervene in a way that might allow everyone a chance to be seen, heard and loved. There was no one with enough wisdom or discernment (or courage) to lean in and embrace the suckiness of it all in the hopes of setting the family free. While I will not minimize or justify their behaviors, the truth is they didn't know there was a better way.

As far as I knew then and as far as I know now (based on conversations with family), no one was talking about how to fix the problem(s). No one was setting up the next generation to know better, to do better. In fact, it was getting worse.

When patterns of behavior and/or beliefs persist from generation to generation, it sets up future generations for more of the same. ***We repeat what we don't repair.*** I would go so far as to say it sets each generation up for worse outcomes.

In Transgenerational Epigenetic Inheritance, particularly when it comes to trauma, what remains unaddressed and unhealed in the generation before allows for the traumatic response to be sort of coded into the expression of the DNA in the next generation and beyond. Without some specific interventions and a nurturing environment, those responses are virtually inevitable. Toxic behaviors and beliefs about ourselves and others are in part, formed and strengthened by the actions of those who have the greatest influence in our childhood. And if we experience first-hand trauma(s) and develop our own trauma responses as a result, it can be the perfect storm that amplifies the destructive outcomes for us and the generations after us.

As for how we can add or subtract to someone's healing journey, connection seems to rule the day. What we know about us humans and how we heal seems to point to a need for true connection and belonging in order for healing and growth to happen. The shame and isolation that come from people passing judgment or providing a rolling commentary from the cheap seats on how much we don't have our act together deepens the divide in relationships and emphasizes the dichotomy between who we're created to be and how we're actually living.

There's a self-perpetuating, self-destructive cycle that occurs when we're steeped in shame. We make internal agreements with ourselves about our value, or lack thereof. We seek out relationships that are in line with

the low value we place on ourselves. We self-medicate and numb. We settle for counterfeit connection which leaves us longing at best and deeply wounded at worst.

When shame is a part of the foundation that we build our life and identity upon, it has the power to determine our ceiling. The experiences of the previous generations can cause us to believe we are unworthy of the good and healthy things in this life. We settle, or worse yet, we set ourselves up to fail, believing failure is inevitable.

But when there's connection? When there's love, acceptance, empathy, forgiveness and grace? Those are the healing elements that nurture us back to health. They allow us to feel safe to explore who we are and to deal with what's happened to us. They can even give us the courage to explore what we've done to ourselves and others that has brought harm. And when we're safely enveloped in relationships where we are seen and reminded of our value and the good that is in us? That's when real change, growth and healing can happen. That's when we break through our ceiling of destructive cycles; where we can believe, embrace and pursue more in this life. That is where shame is slayed, and freedom is found, and where we find who we are truly made to be.

A STRIKING RESEMBLANCE

In hindsight, I wonder what it must've been like for my adopted grandmother, Julie, to have a feisty little reminder of her half-sister Marie living under the same roof as her. I can't help but wonder if she ever projected any of her resentment on to me. Because, sometimes, I swear I could feel it. There were times when it seemed my presence brought her joy, and other times, deep sorrow.

Take for example, the Halloween I was nine and wanted to dress up like a gypsy. Judy did my makeup and adorned my arms and neck with tons

of costume jewelry that weighed me down to the point of discomfort. It was fabulous! And I refused to part with even one bead! She dressed me in a wonderful floral and paisley print, floor-length boho dress with the cutest little go-go boots.

To complete my gypsy ensemble, I borrowed a fiery red wig from Grandma (Julie) and tied a scarf embellished with sequins over the top of the faux hair. I loved my look! Beaming with pride over my super-cool hippie chick gypsy costume, I raced into the kitchen to show Julie. But when she saw me, she burst into tears, and choked out barely audible words. In a gush of air, she exclaimed, "She looks just like Marie!" then ran from the room with her hands over her face.

I was so confused. Who was Marie? Yes, I actually had to ask that question! That's how little the family talked about things. How little they talked about her—my biological grandmother.

Judy had to remind me that Marie was Julie's younger sister, but then quickly changed the subject. She too was upset, but I think more with Julie for upsetting me and forcing her to answer questions she didn't want to answer. I didn't know what to do. So, I did what I always did when people around me weren't okay and I needed them to be. I danced around and made everyone laugh. But I didn't wear the wig. In fact, I can't remember if I even went out for Halloween that year.

MORE ON CHAOS

To my adopted grandmother's (Julie's) credit, having lost her husband a few years before and now having her adult, alcoholic son (Corky), her daughter (Judy) with an ever-growing dependency on pills and alcohol and grand-daughter (me) in her home, she took the role of "matriarch" to a new level.

Julie was what we refer to in counseling as an "over-functioner," also known as an enabler. She ruled the home with an iron hand. Staunchly Catholic, she used God as one of her weapons to keep us all in line, leaving a wake of guilt and shame in all our lives.

If I got into trouble and Judy punished me, it was never harsh enough for Julie—until it was too harsh. Then Julie would swoop in and be my rescuer. If Judy wanted to date, it was forbidden unless Julie approved. If Corky wanted to attempt life on his own, Julie had a thousand reasons why he would never make it. If I did something that was "off" in her opinion, she was quick to point to the picture of Jesus on the wall. "Jesus is watching you," she would say in a deep, ominous voice. This was no ordinary depiction of the Messiah. Not the compassionate, contemplative-faced Jesus at the Last Supper, or holding children on His holy knee. Instead, this was an artist's depiction of the face of The Lord. His eyes masterfully drawn concealing an optical illusion that, once recognized, could not be unseen. Once you gazed upon the closed eyes of Jesus for more than a second, His eyes would suddenly appear to open! Then you could never see them as closed again. Once they opened, they were always open. And as grandma Julie reminded me, always watching. She made it seem as though this was some spiritual mystery of the painting, rather than the talents of a creative (though slightly twisted) artist. Not to mention that no one ever told me we can't actually know what Jesus looked like for sure. From our family's perspective, that painting was as accurate as a photograph.

And so, Jesus, with His watchful, judgy-eyes, became more Boogie Man to me than merciful Savior. I knew He was just waiting for my missteps, for a chance to smite me. And because He didn't seem to take note of the behaviors of anyone else in the family, I decided He was not a god to be trusted. It never occurred to me that Grandma Julie had it all wrong. It also hadn't occurred to me that this was the same version of Jesus she had Judy and Corky believe in as well.

Judy and Corky must have felt like they were suffocating living under their mother's thumb. I was only a small child and I remember feeling like I was suffocating in her presence. We all walked around on egg-shells for fear of igniting each other, each of us trapped in our own little powder keg. Little by little I retreated into myself. This didn't seem to be a problem for anyone in the home. I think everyone was too wrapped up in their own pain to recognize mine.

The elephants in the room were either buried or medicated. Eventually, I would begin to medicate my pain, too.

Judy's abuse of substances worsened. She would have these "spells" where she would get almost catatonic. Her speech would slur, and she would become stiff as a board, barely able to walk or move on her own. Sometimes it would take Julie and Corky together to get her to bed. Other times, Julie would handle it on her own with my help. But never, ever do I remember anyone talking about it the next day. Even when an episode would result in hospitalization. Judy would simply check herself out the next morning, go to work (or home to sleep) and we'd all be there together when I got home from school as if nothing happened.

I remember as a child, looking around the breakfast table, sometimes in Judy's absence, waiting for someone to talk about what had happened. Explain it. Tell me everything was going to be all right or at least tell me where she was. Making a promise that it would never happen again would've been wonderful. Or someone finding the courage to throw the damn pills away. Make her get some help.

But that never happened. Julie would simply call in to Judy's work for her, sighting some unfortunate illness or event that prevented Judy's attendance at work that day and we would resume life as if we were a healthy, happy family. Nothing to see here, folks. Move along.

It was all incredibly frightening and quite frankly, crazy-making for me, a child looking for stability and attempting to rationalize and make sense of it all. I was frantically searching for a way to gain some control over the situation. I thought medications were meant to help a person, yet I knew that she was taking too many and it didn't seem right that she would take them with alcohol. But I didn't know addiction was a legacy in our family and I didn't know there was so much pain and shame at the root of her behaviors. But I did notice that when I was difficult, as children often are, and when things were tense between us or I had trouble at school, she would drink more.

So, I decided the problem was me and I worked hard to be better, to not be so difficult, or ask questions. I did my best not to need parenting. To get perfect grades. I didn't mind sitting on the couch with Judy and Julie, quietly for hours while they watched soap operas, or Sonny and Cher. I Got You, Babe.

Instead of parenting in real life, I found parental guidance for how to live life from TV shows. After all, they seemed to have a better life than I did. There weren't many kids in those shows, but the ones who were seemed to grow up overnight. So, I worked hard to not be a kid, and to grow up overnight too.

My life became about keeping Judy happy and safe, which was really about keeping myself safe, emotionally and physically. As I mentioned earlier, she and Julie shared a bedroom, and I can remember often asking to stay in there with them. Not because I really wanted to, but because on multiple occasions, I could hear Julie yelling at Judy for falling asleep with a lit cigarette hanging out of her mouth exclaiming, "You're going to burn the whole damn house down!"

So, I stayed in the room and waited for her to fall asleep, so I could take the cigarette from her and put it out safely. I learned fast not to be too

eager to take the cigarette. If Judy wasn't asleep and I jumped the gun, there was hell to pay.

The truth is there was almost always some sort of "hell to pay" with Judy, whether it was with me or Corky or even her mother, Julie. I remember the horrible fights Judy and Corky would get into—screaming obscenities at each other, threatening to stab each other with forks. Or knives. Throwing things at each other. Out of fear, I often resorted to attempts at controlling the situation through any means of distraction necessary. One time, the fighting got so bad and I was so afraid that I decided to do something desperate. Swinging between two countertops I let go and fell hard on the wooden floor. With the breath knocked out of me and a searing pain jolting up my spine, everyone froze in place, assuming a cease fire. I got in trouble for my reckless behavior, but at least the fighting and threats had stopped. Brother and sister banded together to make sure I was OK, and to chastise my foolish actions. Externally, some order was momentarily restored. But the chaos raged on inside of me.

YOUR TURN: Reflect. Engage. Write.

Dear Friend, this might be a good place to take a small detour with the part of my story that resonated most deeply with your own. Like most children at this age, I experienced an inappropriate level of agency and believed I had more power to fix things than I actually did. That's why when things went wrong for the adults I loved, I would often think things like, "If only I had been more obedient" or "If I'd kept my room clean."

That, coupled with the adults in my life expecting me to take responsibility for their wellbeing, put me in a position to most often feel that if things were going wrong, it was my fault. And that lie set me up for all sorts of relational dysfunction later in life.

> If you too had an experience in childhood similar to mine, where you knew things were wrong but you couldn't quite figure out what was wrong, and you ended up internalizing the strife and blaming yourself for it, regular talk therapy may fall short in helping you process it. This might be because the emotion/memory/feeling is more visceral than cognitive. What I mean by that is while your mind may struggle to recall details of certain traumatic experiences in your life, you can hold somatic memories (based in the body rather than in the mind) of what occurred. Sometimes, taking a cognitive approach and simply trying to "think differently" about it or process it verbally may not be enough.
>
> The resulting emotions and beliefs from those experiences may be "stuck" in your body, requiring a different form of therapy such as EMDR (which I highly recommend and will explain in more detail later in the book). It was instrumental in my journey. EMDR is a therapy I use with my clients and one I have returned to in my own personal journey on several occasions, including some of the experiences I had while writing this book. In Part Ten, I will go into more detail on this particular therapy as well as some other therapy options to help you decide what might be the best fit for you if you decide to enter into relationship with a trained therapist.
>
> If you have begun to recognize some places in your own story where you would like to experience more awareness and healing, take a moment to write them in your journal now.

HOPE FOR JUDY

With me busy about the business of raising myself and everyone else busy about the business of numbing their own pain, I hardly noticed when slowly, Judy seemed to get "better." She wasn't home as much, which meant she wasn't yelling or taking pills or drinking, so that was good.

But I also noticed that every time Judy came home from being out, while she was in a really good mood, Julie was in a really bad one. Tight faced and scolding, I would hear her say things like "It just isn't right!" and "You'll regret it!" But Judy would ignore her and go about her business. I had no idea what the problem was. And I didn't really care. All I knew was that for the first time in forever, Judy was being an attentive and even fun mom. And I was loving it!

Then one day, I realized what the fuss was all about. Judy had met a man. His name was Bill. He was kind and funny and handsome.

And *Mormon*.

I didn't really know what that meant at the time, but I knew that Julie wasn't having any of it and made several attempts at putting a parental foot down. Still, Judy didn't seem to care. She was smitten with him. It wouldn't be long before I was, too.

She and Bill took me to dinners and to play with his horses. We went to the zoo, movies and shopping; and for the first time in a long time I felt like I was a part of something. *A family.* I felt less like I needed to take care of Judy and more like she was caring for me. She was OK which meant that I was OK. More importantly, for the first time in a long time I felt hope. I think she felt it, too.

Their relationship moved rather quickly and it wasn't long before Bill proposed to Judy. I was so excited! It had been my secret wish and I couldn't believe it was coming true! I can remember wanting that to happen more than I had wanted anything in a long time—maybe ever.

Julie was furious. But for the first and only time that I can remember, Corky was adamantly on his sister's side.

Still, if Julie had anything to say about it, she wasn't going to let her daughter, grown or not, marry a Mormon. Let alone *become* one. The truth was that in her heart of hearts, Judy had no desire to convert either. She talked to Bill, hoping that he would be willing to convert to Catholicism. But in the end, he chose his religion over her. And in my young mind, that meant he chose it over us. Six months later, he was married to another woman.

HOPE LOST

Hindsight being what it is, I can trace the beginning of the end for Judy back to the heartbreak she felt over losing Bill. It was a rapid downhill journey from there. More pills. More drinking. She pulled away as a mom and I retreated back into self-protection and self-sufficiency. But I worked less at protecting her. I held so much anger and disappointment, I no longer cared. I knew what to do for me. And that's what I focused on.

Throughout my childhood, I continued to work hard on my grades and to be as likeable as possible. But when that didn't seem to help me get my needs met or get the attention I so desperately craved, I began to look for other ways to get it and I didn't care if it was in negative or positive ways. I was so tired of being ignored. My soul was starving for attention and affection.

If Julie ever realized just how heartbroken and devastated her daughter was, she certainly never let on. She merely continued to cover up for Judy and her substance abuse. Julie went on as though Bill had never been in the picture. Judy's parenting ability declined even further and the more Julie tried to step in and parent me in her place, the more I rebelled. I wanted answers as to why this man I had hung so many hopes on was no longer a part of our lives. But I don't recall any conversations about the breakup either. Like most people who disappeared from our

lives, because of a relationship that ended or a death, he was never talked about again.

BREAKING A CHILD'S HEART

In my constant quest for belonging, I joined the Girl Scouts when I was nine. Little did I know that decision would usher in one of the deepest heartbreaking experiences of my life. On one particular domestically-focused outing, my troop was given the opportunity to bake and decorate cakes like professional bakers. I'm not talking a little icing and sprinkles on a box-mix cake. I'm talking made-from-scratch-cake and icing adorned with full-blown *Cake Boss* type decorations. Or, at least in my little, 9-year-old mind, that's what my confectionary creation looked like.

As luck would have it, that week in October was Judy's birthday, so I was doubly excited to give her the gift of my one-of-a-kind creation. I carried it with such caution, you would've thought I was transporting explosives! I could hardly contain my excitement as I waited for her to get home from work.

In my exuberance, I didn't really notice that something was off in her demeanor when she walked through the door. Perhaps I thought that whatever it might be, my magical cake would make her forget all about it.

Judy wasn't completely through the door when I sprang from my perch on the couch in front of the big picture window. "Happy Birthday Mom!" And before she could respond, I rapidly began detailing the process of making the cake as I dragged her into the kitchen to see the masterpiece with her own eyes.

"MOM! I can't believe the luck! I got to make this for you on your BIRTHDAY! All the other kids had to come up with some sort of theme for their cakes but when I said mine was for your birthday, they let me create whatever cake I thought you would want. Isn't that cool?!"

I was practically singing my words, rambling with excitement. I made sure she paid special attention to the writing on the cake **"HApPy BIrtH-dAY MoM."** I told her about the flavors we used and how I just knew she was going to love it. She kept trying to talk over me, to interject a word in edgewise, but I would not be deterred. She managed a weak smile but dismissed most of what I was saying. She was tired and all she really wanted was for me to help make dinner. But I wanted her to eat dessert first.

"Just try it, Mom," I begged trying to reach a small plate from the cabinet overhead. Julie kindly took one down and handed it to me so I could hand it to Judy.

"Later, Gina. I'm tired. We need dinner first." She said through gritted teeth.

"Mom, haha, I *knooooow* we do! But just try it! Grandma, tell her to try it!" I protested.

Julie just smiled and shook her head.

Judy repeated her insistence that we cook dinner, and I rebutted, determined to make her smile and Eat. The. Cake. I just knew all would be well if she would just *Eat. The. Cake.* Even Julie seemed in favor of cake over dinner in that moment. While Julie and I were distracted by our laughter and my protests, neither one of us were able to head off the explosion set to blow from Judy.

Suddenly, *WHACK!* With one smooth, ninja-like move, Judy swept the cake off the countertop and slammed it, upside down into the garbage can.

Time froze. I couldn't breathe. My brain refused to accept what just happened. The three of us stood there, each with a look of utter shock on our faces. In hindsight, I think Judy shocked herself as much as she did me. Julie gasped. Then shouted *"Oh, Judy! What did you do?"*

But it was too late. My heart was smashed, just like the cake. I had dared to trust, dared to reach out, dared to connect and it went horribly wrong. My childish heart somehow believed for a moment that this cake could somehow heal all the brokenness in our lives. It was too much to expect. I felt so much shame in that moment. So much disappointment. The reality of who we all were wickedly mocking my attempts at becoming something more.

I know Judy felt terrible. She even attempted to dig to the middle of the cake and find a bite she could take that hadn't been contaminated by coffee grounds and eggshells discarded from breakfast that morning. But it was too late. The cake couldn't be salvaged. Neither could my belief that it would be safe to expose my heart, or my hope that she could be trusted to be the mother I needed her to be. The damage was done.

When Judy produced her thimble full of clean cake from the waste basket, I offered a weak smile and pretended to feel better when she said the cake was really good. Something had already shut down in me that day. I didn't consciously realize it in the moment, but later in life as I worked through my story, that memory surfaced time and time again and I realized that day was a significant turning point in my life.

My experience that day confirmed a message that seemed to be repeating. One that would continue to replay—I needed to put an end to the child in me. Much like those around me, I resented her for needing, for

not being able to care completely for herself. I hated her for hoping. For trusting. I think I hated her for needing love. The vulnerability of my child-self compromised my safety and I knew that had to change. Quickly.

YOUR TURN: Reflect. Engage. Write.

Dear Friend, perhaps you have already recognized the implications of my emotional shut down that day. Maybe you have felt something similar?

In the incident with the cake, and perhaps in several moments over the years leading up to that day, I had made a decision that I couldn't trust anyone with the most vulnerable parts of me. I couldn't trust those charged with my care to give me what I needed in this life and I was going to need to figure out how to get it for myself. In a sense I decided that while surrounded by many people, I was alone. Eventually, when your greatest hopes and cries for connection and belonging go unanswered, you simply stop asking. But the need for it doesn't go away.

That time in my life set off a confusing and dark spiral. I had no idea just how much darker it would get before I would find the Light. Or should I say, before the Light found me.

If this portion of the story has called to mind anything specific in your own story, this would be good time to journal those thoughts. They might lead you to places where you made unhealthy and unhelpful agreements with yourself that now need to be broken.

CHAPTER 8 Hoping for Hope

A REFUGE LOST

As my home life disintegrated, the teachers at school (mostly nuns) treated me more and more like a pariah, some going so far as to tell the parents of my friends that I was from a "broken home," and they would do their best to keep their kids from going to my home or hanging out with me. The more friends at school told me this, the more it confirmed the shame I already carried. Soon, I began to avoid teachers, too, and my grades started to fall. It wasn't long before most of my interactions with faculty were negative ones. I began to feel the same way at school that I did at home. Although the two worlds rarely converged until one day when I was 10.

As lunch period began, I was distractedly walking to the cafeteria, consumed by the events of my math class the period before where incessant prodding from a "friend" convinced me to share my answers with her. I feared being labeled a cheater and felt sick to my stomach. I was just getting into line when I was called out by the principal. *"Here we go,"* I thought, just wondering what punishment was in store.

Sister Agnus walked alongside me with an uncharacteristically gentle look on her face. Which, of course, made me immediately suspicious. By that age, I had become very good at reading people, and I began to realize her countenance didn't fit with someone about to deliver a punishment.

As we walked through the double doors into the hallway, my Uncle Corky was standing there; a look was on his face that was difficult to read, even for me. He seemed despondent and panic rose within me, although I was uncertain as to why.

"I came to bring you home," was all he said. His voice sounding sort of disconnected. Robotic.

"Oh, ...OK..." I responded with trepidation. He didn't say much on the way home, and the silence was uncomfortable. I attempted to make small talk to fill the anxious void, but he wouldn't engage. Clearly *something* was wrong. Per the usual, fearing it was something I had done wrong, I set about the business of attempting to make it right. But when we got home, Judy's car was parked in front as well as Ernie's. I couldn't imagine what would bring them together, but I feared it was something terrible. Uncle Corky told me to wait while he went in the kitchen, so I dutifully stood by the overstuffed chair, just inside the front door, like an outsider waiting to be invited into the fold.

It felt like forever, but only a moment passed before he summoned me into the kitchen. As I came around the corner, my sense that something was horribly wrong was confirmed by Judy's red, swollen eyes and the sorrowful look on Ernie's face. I don't remember who said it first, but I think it was Ernie. He told me that my grandmother, Julie, had died.

"How is that possible?" I thought. *"I just saw her this morning."* I wanted to ask questions, to express my confusion. I wanted to argue and say it wasn't possible. But I had no words. No one else did either. I just

quietly retreated to my room. I don't remember how long I stayed there, tending to myself, before anyone checked on me. Perhaps I came out on my own.

I don't remember anyone talking to me about it beyond telling me it happened. But I do recall the feeling of complete disconnection, like everyone was walking around in the same room with walls around them that no one could get through. All of us alone, together. Tears with no comfort offered. Grief unshared. Pain undivided. No one to help hold the weight of it all.

The more time passed the more questions raced through my mind, but none that I dared to vocalize. What were we going to do now? What would happen to us? How was I going to survive with Judy and Corky? Who would break up fights? Who would tell my mom what to do? What would happen when she had one of her "spells?" As I think back on it now and recognize the giant hole it is in my memory, it's a clear example of a time when I dissociated. (For those who don't know, dissociation is a sort of 'trick of the mind' in which the mind separates itself and our emotions from the physical world in order to protect us from things we simply cannot process in a healthful way. Dissociation explains a lot of the holes in my narrative. If you have holes in your narrative, perhaps it explains them for you as well.)

It may come as no surprise that I don't really remember Julie's funeral. I just remember no one really talked about her again once it was over. I don't recall anyone asking me how I was or what I was feeling. Just like every other person who had died in the family before her, when you're gone, you're gone. It seemed almost expected that you would deal with it in your own way. In many ways, it felt like we were encouraged to forget.

All I can remember thinking was, *"If I die or leave, will I be forgotten too?"*

FINDING CONNECTION

As I said, I don't remember much about Julie's funeral. And yet, those days of the visitation and burial were lifechanging for me. Although not in the way you might be thinking.

A very special person attended all three days of the funeral, along with her husband. This woman was wonderful in so many ways. She was warm and kind, funny (yes, even at a funeral home) and larger than life. She was also very pretty, with piercing green eyes and a contagious laugh. She seemed to light up the dark and solemn funeral home while simultaneously setting off a wave of whispers amidst looks of shock and awe from many members of my extended family. All of which admittedly made her even more appealing to me.

Many in attendance were happy to see her—the light she illuminated brightened the darker countenance of some in her presence. Then there were others who were whispering, and mobbing Judy and Ernie to discuss this mystery woman's presence. But that didn't deter me from wanting to know her and be near her. After all, I was used to whispers and secrets.

I felt an instant connection to this mystery woman, and I deeply wanted to know her. I waited impatiently for someone to introduce me, but everyone seemed overly interested in occupying my time with other things to distract me. And all that unusual "attention" made me suspicious.

And *irritated.*

Finally, I saw a break in the sea of people around me and beelined for this woman. While I can't remember exactly what each of us said, I do remember what I *felt*: her warmth and instant affection for me. And as crazy as it may sound, I felt the same thing for her. If I close my eyes, I can almost see the small, floral couch in the cramped parlor area.

Without waiting for permission, I squeezed myself in between her and the arm of the worn sofa, tucking myself in tight. Before too many words could pass between us, Judy and a few other relatives were there, interrupting the conversation in order to make a proper introduction.

"Gina, this is your cousin Cathy," Judy said. Ernie was standing behind her with a look of irritation on his face. For the first time in maybe forever, I knew that look wasn't directed at me. It seemed as though it was actually in my favor.

But the look on Judy's face? *That* look was directed at Cathy. It appeared Judy was communicating volumes without speaking a word in the way only Judy could. None of it friendly. I'm certain a complete stranger would have felt the tension. And yet I remained undeterred and did not budge from my post.

I really wanted Cathy to like me, so I was bright and bubbly—somewhat out of place for a funeral home. "Nice to meet you!" I said, sticking my hand out for a proper shake like the adults did, even though I had been sitting there a solid ten minutes prior.

"Nice to meet you, too," she said softly, giving first my hand, and then my shoulders a gentle squeeze. I thought I saw tears glistening at the corners of her eyes but didn't think much of it. We were at a funeral home after all.

Over the course of those three days, I packed in as much interaction with Cathy as possible; savoring every moment of her affection and attention. It was a precious respite from my homelife and what would certainly be the devastating aftermath from Julie's death.

Sadly, Cathy's husband didn't seem very interested in our new relationship, but I was too enamored with Cathy to care. Still, I could feel his disapproving gaze often, so I just avoided him.

The day of the burial came and with it, my need to say goodbye to this new and very special relative. Truth be told, and as crazy as it might sound, I think I grieved the idea of not seeing Cathy again more than Julie's death. At least at the time I did.

As Cathy and I said our goodbyes, I felt an inexplicable depth of sorrow and I cried my eyes out. For reasons unknown to me, she cried too. But as we said our final farewell, Cathy leaned in close and squeezed me tight. "We *will* see each other again, sweetheart. I promise." And for some reason, I completely believed her. She gave me one final kiss on the head and said, "I love you." Then, she got in her car with her husband and drove away. But a part of her stayed right there, tucked safely away in my heart.

That night, and for many nights to follow, I couldn't get her out of my mind. What she gave me in those three short days was what my heart had so deeply longed for. It was like fresh rain on a parched land. And it was glorious. And I wanted more of it. I longed to see her again. I talked about her incessantly. It drove Judy crazy. So I decided to cool it around her, but my mind continued to fantasize about hanging out with Cathy again. Fortunately, I was able to talk about her at Ernie's. He didn't seem to mind at all.

As time passed, I thought about her a little less. But she was never farther than the back of my mind. I never stopped hoping for the day when I could see her again.

While it was a sweet time of connection for Cathy and me, it took my attention away from the loss of Julie, which was both good and bad. Because there would be no opportunity to process it with anyone later, I think I lost the opportunity to fully grieve Julie's death. Not that I would have known how to truly grieve anyway. While the time and place of our interactions made the connection complicated, that love and acceptance was a definite blessing.

SOMEHOW, YOU JUST *KNOW*

Up to this point in my life, the subject of my adoption had only surfaced a handful of times. I don't recall a "first time," as in, someone sitting me down and explaining the whole thing. It was as if it was just assumed I knew, no differently than one would assume I knew the color of my own eyes. For the most part, it was treated as an off-limits conversation (My adoption. Not the color of my eyes.) Judy and Ernie preferred pretending it didn't really happen and typically, I saw no reason to push the subject, so I didn't bring it up much.

Then, one day at school, a teacher read a story about a young boy who was adopted, and I made the grave error of telling my classmates, who already saw me as an outcast (remember, "broken home") that like the character in our story, I too was adopted. Their teasing was immediate and relentless.

"So, you don't know who your parents *really* are?" One girl taunted. It didn't take long for the rest of my "friends" to join in the jeers and taunting.

"I do too!" I shouted in my most defiant tone. In that moment, my mind was grasping for something to make the teasing stop. But the next words that left my mouth shocked me as much as my classmates. It was as though they were spoken from somewhere outside myself, not fully resonated in my brain before I heard them with ears. "I do know who they are! My *real* mom's name is Cathy!"

While my proud proclamation silenced the bullies, the voices inside my mind were rapidly repeating the words I had just said. I knew I had chosen the woman from the funeral because there was a part of me that wished she were my mother. But what if it were true?

"Could that be right?" I thought to myself. *"That woman at the funeral, Cathy! Could she really be my mom?"* The thought distracted me all day. And the next. And the next. It stayed with me, a constant secret companion. I dared not mention it to Judy.

The more I thought about Cathy and the way everyone behaved at the funeral, the more my fantasy became plausible.

The truth is I had this wonder and hope almost immediately after meeting her. But I didn't dare allow myself to entertain such an incredible notion for more than a second. But now it felt almost certain. I knew I had to proceed very carefully, fearing if I said the wrong thing to the wrong person, it would destroy my chances of ever seeing her again. It seemed my only hope of finding the truth was with Ernie. But how would I tell him what I already knew—that Cathy was my mother?

ERNIE HAD A SECRET TOO

While time passed, I hadn't let go of my belief that Cathy was my biological mom. In fact, I spent an unhealthy amount of time imagining, hoping and dreaming that she was my mother. I became obsessed with knowing if the words I blurted out that day at school were as true as I believed them to be.

I was still spending every other weekend with Ernie, welcomed breaks from the chaos of my home with Judy and Corky. On an especially good weekend with Ernie, after he and Judy had yet another knock down drag out fight, I decided the timing was perfect for me to muster up the courage to ask him about Cathy. I knew the timing was right to ask, but I struggled to find my "in."

Friday night came and went. Saturday did the same. By Saturday evening, I was certain I had lost my nerve. But then Sunday morning came

and over frosted flakes and sausage (a typical breakfast with Dad), I let my question fly in one garbled mess of words and breath.

"Hey Dad, I need to ask you a question." (No pause for response.) "I'm wondering if that Cousin Cathy person I met at Grandma Julie's funeral is my *real* mom." I held my breath and studied his face for a reaction. Surprisingly, he seemed relatively unfazed.

"I think you already know the answer to that question, babe. Don't you?" His voice was gentle, and completely void of any anxiousness you might expect him to feel when faced with such a question.

But, what the hell kind of answer was that?

He was notorious for making me think that things I had heard or seen weren't *really* real. He worked hard and mostly failed at keeping secrets from me and when he failed, he just insisted, emphatically, that I had mis-seen, misheard, or misread the circumstances or person in question. And if I insisted that I knew what I had seen, heard, read, then I was the one in trouble. So, while I was certain that I knew what I knew about Cathy, I was uncertain if it was OK to know it. Not sure how to respond to him, I just sort of froze.

Fortunately, Ernie read my panic and confusion. His face softened and he told me that I was correct. He didn't say much more than that. His reaction was as though I had asked some simple question with a simple answer. Like I had just asked him if the table was made of wood or something. Or if the sun was shining.

I was wondering if that would be the end of it. There was no conversation. No explanation. No mention of getting to see her again. Instead, Ernie told me he was going to call his friend Charlie (the one he called every Sunday evening for a chat) and we could talk later. This meant I had to leave the room. For some reason, I always had to leave the room

when he talked to Charlie. Ernie gently sent me away with my confusion and frustration for a little TV distraction.

Like a good girl, I obeyed and went into the living room at the other end of the house. Fortunately for me, one of my favorite distractions was on—*Wonder Woman.* I had just settled into my television escape when Ernie called me back into the kitchen.

Energized by the intro to the show, I took the superhero route to the kitchen, through the shotgun style floorplan of the apartment, running as fast as I could across the wooden floors in my socked feet, then sliding onto the kitchen tile, poised for battle.

I made my abrupt stop at the kitchen table where Ernie sat with his back to me, curled over the phone as though he was protecting it from something. The receiver still in his hand, he looked at me with more uncertainty than I'd ever seen on his face. We both just sort of stalled there. Neither of us sure what should come next.

"Hey Kiddo. You know my friend Charlie here, right?" he said, pointing to the receiver. I shook my head "yes," but the truth was, I didn't really *know* Charlie. I mean, sure they talked whenever I was there on Sundays. But I never got on the phone with him. Sometimes Ernie would tell me to shout out a "Hi Charlie" or have me sing a song I recently learned in choir (which I thought was a little odd, but I never passed up the chance to entertain someone and make them happy). But I didn't really "know" Charlie.

Finally, I answered "Sure, Dad" because it was just easier.

"Well, I need to tell you something about Charlie. 'Charlie' is really more of nickname. And Charlie is more than just a friend of mine. She is part of the family. Charlie is really Cathy, your biological mom. She would like to talk to you if you want to talk to her. Here ya go."

And with that, he simply handed me the phone.

What I remember most in those moments was the shock and how surreal it all felt. I was happy, but I had so many questions in that moment. None that would be answered then, or even later. No time to process what had just happened. Confusion overwhelmed me and I think I disconnected a bit. There were so many questions rolling around in my head. (Later in life, more questions came.) But in that moment, I fought hard to stay present. I had waited for what felt like forever to talk with her again. I didn't want to miss a second of it.

I wish I could remember exactly what happened next. But I can't fully recall the details. Time sort of stood still. I can remember what it felt like in my body though. I was positively giddy, and a little sick to my stomach as I often became when things were intensely emotional. I've learned over time that deeply emotional memories can be like that; our minds may not recall the exact circumstances, but our bodies can recall the feelings, sometimes more than we want them to.

My stomach flip-flopped, my heart raced. I remember crying. And I remember her crying too. I remember talking to her about wanting to see her again. She assured me we would figure it out. I had so much I wanted to say to her, but I was having a hard time getting my words out.

It felt like I was only on the phone with her for a second before Ernie was telling me to give the phone back. And I remember being so afraid to let go of the receiver—afraid to take it from my ear. The warmth of it against my head and her soft voice coming through felt like a vaguely familiar connection of safety and I really didn't want to let it go.

I can't fully recall how our conversation ended but I do remember her telling me she loved me. I reflexively said it back, but I think I meant it too. I was a bit too young to entertain all the questions that would come

later regarding her love for me, and how we can only give love out of what we have. Sometimes what we have is brokenness.

After the call, I remember asking Ernie over and over again when I could talk to her next. Could she come over and get me? Could we go see her? Didn't she say at the funeral that she had sons? If she has sons, then they would be my *brothers*, right?! Is her husband my *real* dad? (I would imagine that question hurt Ernie, but that was not my intention.) I'm sure my barrage of questions made Ernie second guess his decision to tell me about Cathy in the way he did. But I'd like to think his motives for doing so were good. While I really did want answers to my questions, I was mostly giving voice to some of my dreams about what it would be like if she were my mom, and what it would be like for those dreams to come true. But above all else, I really just wanted to see her again.

That opportunity would come soon enough. Cathy would make sure of that. She was as eager to see me as I was to see her.

But first, Ernie had to tell Judy what he had done. Apparently, telling me about Cathy was not a joint decision. Fortunately for me, the conversation about it took place between the two of them on the street while I was in the house putting my things away. Despite the distance I could hear their raised voices and the occasional curse word. Peeking through the curtains, I could see Judy's flailing arms as she jabbed a scolding, pointy finger in Ernie's face. I fully expected I would get into trouble as well once he was gone, but I think she sensed there was no undoing what had been done.

MEETING CATHY AGAIN

Judy put her anger aside and it wasn't long before arrangements were made for me to see Cathy and her family. *My* family. The adults made the plan and, on a Friday after school, Cathy and her husband David picked me up from a friend's house where I would occasionally wait for

Judy to get off of work. Apparently, Judy had no interest in being near Cathy. As for Ernie, I'm not sure why he decided against being there. But there I was, with my friend and her parents. Judy had packed me an overnight bag, somehow comfortable with the idea of me spending the entire weekend with Cathy and David. At 11, I was too young (and too excited!) to see how horribly wrong it had all been handled.

For some reason, it was decided that a public meeting with my half-brothers would be best. So, they had decided we would meet, of all places, at a Jack n' the Box.

"The boys are with family waiting to meet you!" Cathy said in the most chipper of voices. I can only imagine it felt like some of her dreams about having all her children together were coming true.

When we arrived, the place was packed. I remember instantly feeling panic. My face grew hot and my stomach churned. I didn't want all those people there. I didn't have the words at the time, but it felt like a violation, like strangers walking in on the birth of a child.

My anxiety spiked as I realized virtually everyone in the place was staring at me. It was as if they knew why I was there and were waiting for the show to start. I fought the urge to ask Cathy if we could leave.

But quickly it was revealed that all of those eyes were on me for a reason. Virtually everyone in the place (besides the employees and a few unsuspecting customers) were related to Cathy, and consequently, related to me. They were her siblings, sibling-in-laws and their children, my aunts and uncles and cousins and of course, my half-brothers. Everyone wanted in on the reunion. So many people introducing themselves. Cathy introducing "this aunt" and "that uncle." Everyone was hugging me; invading my space, telling me how happy they were to "have me back." Whatever *that* meant. Cathy was crying, tears of joy, I believe. All

the while her husband, David, was standing in the corner with his arms folded over his chest, a reluctant and disgruntled observer.

As well-meaning as the extended family was, it proved too overwhelming for me and as a result, I don't remember much about that portion of the day. I'm confident that's because I dissociated in response to the stress.

It will come as no surprise that further details of that day become sketchy from here. (Just a reminder, *dissociated* is a clinical term for "my emotions were on overload and in order to protect itself, my brain pulled a "peace out." My body was there but my brain sort of packed up my emotions and took a vacay.)

While the specifics are really dim, here's what I do remember. We went to Cathy's stepmom's home (the home she never quite fit into as an adolescent) where I was shown copious amounts of pictures of people who were apparently related to me but for whom I had zero context in terms of where or how they should fit into my life, particularly since a few of them were dead.

And then, there were those three, rambunctious little boys; my brothers. It was kind of cool to be a big sister but, I didn't really have context for them either. They called me "sissy" and seemed happy I was there. But that was probably because I paid attention to them and played with them.

The only issue was that I was getting a whole lot of attention from Cathy that formerly belonged to them and they weren't too happy about that. They were small, so who could blame them? It was clear they were feeling jealous. But again, I can see how they might've felt I was somehow a threat, even though they wouldn't have had words for that either. Oh, and they were mischievous! Which was *also* familiar. A trait that revealed heredity.

Within a couple of hours, they did the typical things little brothers do. They started going through my overnight bag. As my new little brothers

were pilfering through my things, they came across my makeup bag and began dumping it out. *(Yep, I was probably too young for a makeup bag, but I was in a terrible hurry to grow up.)*

In all fairness to them, they didn't know what to do with a big sister and all the trappings that came with her. And to be fair to me, I had no idea what to do with all those cute, grubby little hands rummaging through my treasures! I thrived on being in control in order to be safe, and I did not feel in control.

It wasn't but a heartbeat before they found my liquid foundation and opened the bottle, turning it upside down to see if it would pour out of the bottle. Which it did. All over my clothes. The ones I had so carefully selected so I would look my best for my first weekend with my mother. I wanted so much to impress her and make her proud to be seen with me. I needed everything to go perfectly so she would want to see me again, and makeup all over my clothes was seriously messing with my plan. So I did what any insecure young girl with attachment wounds would do. I *freaked* out.

Snatching the bottle, I yelled at them all to "stay out of my stuff!" and before I knew it, David, Cathy's husband, was there, snatching the makeup out of my hand. Putting the lid on the bottle and placing it so high on a shelf even I couldn't reach it. With venom in his words, he gently picked up my brothers and shot me a look of anger and disgust as he ushered them away from me.

"Come on boys," he growled, "let's not mess with the princess and her things."

I felt a lot of things in that moment, but I assure you, feeling like a princess was not one of them.

Generations/Family Relationships Chart reference, page 347

YOUR TURN: Reflect. Engage. Write.

Dear Friend, I don't know the story of how my mom met David, but to this day the attraction is a mystery to me. They were as opposite as two people could be. David was a quiet man, introverted and pessimistic, large in frame and form. I remember, he always looked at me as though my very existence was a problem for him. He had this heavy sigh that spoke volumes about the level of disgust and frustration he was feeling about pretty much everything in the world around him that wasn't affiliated with him getting his way. With that one special sigh, he could send my stomach into summersaults and my heart racing.

For as much as I know about how Cathy and David met, I know even less about his history, except to say I do remember meeting his parents once when I was visiting my mom and brothers. They were polite but cold. Perhaps their coldness was the result of me being who I was and all I represented to them, or, perhaps the result of them being them and all that they'd experienced in their own stories. But *most* likely, it was a combination of both.

Perhaps this portion of the story has reminded you of some impactful part of your own story; a part that caused you to feel unwanted or threatened. Maybe my interactions with David and even those with other family members have reminded you of people in your own story. If so, I would encourage you to journal about that now.

CHAPTER 9 Wanting It to Work

AUDITIONING FOR FAMILY

Despite the already unhealthy relationship between David and me, I settled into acceptance that he was my "stepfather" and tried to be outwardly happy about it so that I could spend more time with my biological mom, Cathy, and my little brothers. The school year was ending and I was really hoping to spend some of the summer with Cathy. Unbeknownst to me, she had the same idea and had already been working with Ernie and Judy to arrange for me to spend the *entire* summer at her house. As with all other matters pertaining to Cathy, Ernie was my champion, while Judy was less than thrilled with the idea of me spending so much time with Cathy.

Although she was already distant from the role of "mom" (favoring more of a friendship with me instead), Judy set about finding new ways to engender herself as my favorite. She took me shopping and let me buy short-shorts, tons of makeup, large, dangly earrings and a wardrobe full of other items that would typically be mother-*dis*approved clothing. We went out to eat several times a week leading up to my departure for

Cathy's and on most of our dinner outings, she ramped up the friend game by letting me drink wine at the sophisticated age of 12.

If Judy's goal was to entice me into staying with her, it didn't work. And it wasn't long before I was packing my things for a blissful, three-month stay at Cathy's. I was so excited! Truth be told, I probably had some lofty and unrealistic expectations going into the situation. The reality of it was that it was a mix of good, bad and ugly, almost from the beginning.

The first of the "ugly" came in the form of the first mother/daughter fight between Cathy and me, courtesy of Judy and the short-shorts and makeup which were clearly inappropriate for a 12-year-old girl.

But the good was *really* good. Cathy was affectionate, kind and creative. She inspired me to be creative too. I felt even more like her daughter knowing we shared a love of all things creative; music, writing, drawing, creating in general. With sidewalk chalk or instruments, it all felt like bonding over some sort of special gift we shared.

As I mentioned before, Cathy was hilarious with a contagious laugh and she constantly looked for ways to engage and connect with me that summer. She had decorated a room in the basement for me and even let me pick out the wallpaper—big, bright flowers with tons of pink, purple, orange and green, and sparkly yellow centers that glistened when kissed by light—sort of like Gerber daisies on steroids; before they were the "in thing."

She tried to make it feel like home. Like *my* home. She introduced me to the neighbors and even worked to help me make friends with some of the kids my age in her neighborhood by inviting them over and doing our hair and makeup (age appropriate, of course). She suggested sleep overs and offered to host them as well as camp outs in the back yard.

She encouraged me to bond with my brothers, which admittedly was difficult having been raised as an only child. Cathy even found ways to encourage my relationship with Dave. Including pressing me to call him dad.

She did her best to meld us into one big happy family as though we had always been that way. But none of us had context for each other in those roles in our lives. True to the family way, we didn't talk about the elephant in the room. In all fairness, it is likely that no one would have been able to identify it either. No one advocated for slowing things down and honoring the confusion and possible pain some of us (me) might have been experiencing. I certainly wasn't allowing myself to feel anything other than happy. I was incredibly anxious and unsettled most of the time, but I did whatever I could to push through it, even though it made me physically ill at times. I didn't want to give Cathy any reason to take me back to Judy's.

But all that ignoring and pretending and redirecting finally caught up with us and as hard as most of us tried to make it work, it wasn't long before things started to go wrong.

One of my biggest challenges was with my brothers. Cathy had them calling me "Sissy" before it had fully sunk in that I was, in fact, a "big sister." It was sweet and well-intentioned, I'm sure. However, I had no idea how to be a big sister and for the most part felt like I was in competition with them for my Mom's affection most of the time. I was trying so hard to connect with her, trying to soak in some semblance of motherly nurturing and love. But it seemed like every time I tried to talk to her or just be with her, there was a little brother in my way, either trying to get her attention or mine.

It wasn't that I didn't want *any* connection with them. I did! They were super-cute and a ton of fun. They were also cuddly which worked out well because I *loved* hugs. The oldest of the three was inquisitive, wanting to know everything about me and trying to emulate the things I said and did.

All three of them would do just about anything I told them to, from getting me an extra cookie from the kitchen to painting each other with finger paints instead of the paper, which, in typical big-sister form, made me a little drunk with power.

Despite the fun the boys and I were having, David saw me as real competition for his sons. I think he saw me as competition for himself as well. He went out of his way to stay emotionally removed from me. He would take the boys to do things and leave me out. He would yell, pout and manipulate to pull Cathy away. It didn't matter what I did to try and make him like me. His mind was made up—there was no place for me in his family.

Navigating relationships in their home wasn't the only place I struggled. Things were a bit off with the neighborhood girls, too. The more they learned about my situation, the less they understood my home life. It would have been complicated enough for an adult to comprehend and keep straight who was who in my family and all the dual roles people played ("My cousin is actually my mother?"). It was too much to ask of a gaggle of pre-teen girls. Eventually, endorsed by their parents, they sought distance from me, which reinforced my shame. The only thing I could feel was homesick and defeated. It was all too difficult. I couldn't figure out my role. At least at Judy's I knew how to function within that dysfunction, which felt safer than this new uncertainty.

I didn't last the summer before I was begging to go back to Judy's, with an agreement that we would continue to visit every so often. While I was the one asking to go back home, Cathy was the one who seemed most relieved by my request. David seemed downright elated.

I felt like somehow, I had failed. I wouldn't have had the vocabulary to explain it at the time but looking back I think I felt like I was being given up all over again. I had auditioned for the role of daughter but didn't get the part. My chance to be part of a "real" family was gone and with it all

the fantasies I had held about life with Cathy. A whole new attachment wound was formed. Or perhaps, the existing one was just deepened.

But this time, I made an agreement with myself that I wouldn't dare to hope it could be different in the future. I was through hoping someone would give me the chance to just "be a kid"—to be loved unconditionally. From there I made it my mission to lock away any part of me that remained in childlike dependence on the people around me. The events that summer confirmed something I had started to believe at a very, very young age: *If anyone was going to take care of me, it would need to be me.*

YOUR TURN: Reflect. Engage. Write.

Dear Friend, I'm curious if you can see the patterns beginning to repeat from Cathy's life into mine?

Remember, when she tried to live with her father and stepmother and siblings? It did not go well. Her step-mom remained cold and detached, which eventually contributed to Cathy being forced to move back in with Tony and Lucy.

What do you suppose might have happened if Cathy had told David of her experience and how negatively it affected her life?

What if she determined to not allow him to treat me the way she had been treated?

What else do you see repeating? Are you taking some guesses at what might have helped?

Is any of this helping you think through your own story?

Take some time to reflect and write your answers.

CHAPTER 10 A Darker Spiral

THE LAST OF INNOCENCE LOST

Trigger Warning: if you've had trauma of a sexual nature in your history, please proceed through the following section with caution.

Following my rough summer at Cathy's and at home, the new school year started. I continued to fight against the image of being from a "broken home," so things were unraveling at school, as well. Still, there was space to find some connection and even a sense of worth in my classes, particularly when it came to writing, or anything that required creativity. But the more I experimented with drugs and alcohol and other means of numbing out, the less I felt like I belonged with kids my age.

My new friends, all at least three years older than me, had begun introducing me to all things "mature." I was smoking (all kinds of things), drinking (which wasn't that much of a stretch, considering I'd started drinking with Judy a few months before), and just before my 13th birthday, began to dabble in drugs.

But every once in a while, when I was with kids from school, I would long to be like them, *normal*. I still attempted to fit in. I even started talking with a couple of boys who walked my same route home each day. They were popular and I clearly was not. I figured if I was accepted by them, I might have a shot at being accepted by others.

I branched out in my creativity and began to play guitar and sing several times a month at mass in the mornings (as a student body, we went to church *every* morning before school). This was in direct contradiction with my behaviors outside of school and on more than one occasion, I wondered if I would burst into flames when I approached the alter to sing. I also started hanging out at the convent on our school campus and stayed after for any and every program I could find. I think that singing at church and hanging out with the nuns gave me some sort of hope that I could earn God's favor, that He would protect me; rescue me from my homelife, rescue me from myself. But a person can only lead a double life for so long before one of those lives becomes dominant. I think there was something within me that knew I was on a slippery slope with my new, older friends outside of school. It was like a part of me could sense the impending danger, so I tried to immerse myself in things that kept me with kids my age.

I worked feverishly to fit in and leaned in wherever I was shown attention. I began to crush on a boy in school, who seemed kind and went out of his way to talk to me and be attentive.

He showed up at a friend's pool party one weekend and, while under water, kissed me.

It would've been impossible to keep it a secret though, given both of us breeched the surface with the force of a nuclear missile. We just stared at each other for a moment, our eyes as round as the innertubes floating around the pool. We felt both a mixture of shock and confusion. I quickly swam for the ladder amidst the whispers and giggles of everyone

present. With no conversation on my part, I clamored out as fast as my shame-weakened legs would carry me and practically ran home, dripping all the way.

Once home and alone in my room, I was grateful for the pot hidden beneath my guinea pig's cage. I was so glad it was a Friday! But come Monday, I did not want to go to school. I knew this boy would've told all the other boys and God only knew who else would know.

Imagine my surprise when absolutely nothing was said.

The closer I got to the end of the day, the more I relaxed. As the dismissal bell rang, I gathered my things for the walk home, feeling relieved and happy. *"It's going to be OK,"* I thought. *"It's really going to be OK."*

I was walking home unceremoniously with the usual crew of misguided, fellow delinquents, when about two blocks from school, three of my crush's friends caught up with me. We were just walking and talking, but then, their questioning began. *"What did YOU do this weekend, Gina?"* One boy who had missed the party asked, as the other two jabbed each other in the side with their elbows.

My stomach turned sour and my brain started to buzz. *"They know,"* I thought to myself. But the sensation I felt was more than the fear of them knowing. Something felt...dark. A sense of dread filled my body. I felt the urge to run but couldn't understand why. My legs felt like I was walking in wet cement. I chastised myself for feeling that way. Told myself I was a coward, and I shouldn't run. After all, if I wanted to be friends with these guys, it wouldn't happen by acting crazy. Besides, I had learned to ignore my own feelings, to doubt my experiences and feel shame for being afraid or sad. I had learned to conform to other's needs to be accepted. So, I ignored what my gut was telling me.

The boys started asking questions about me kissing John. "How did it feel?" one asked, sidling up on my left. "I'll bet you liked it," he growled in my ear.

"What base did you let him get to?" asked the other boy, blocking me on the right. I felt trapped between them when suddenly, his hand was down my shirt while the other boy held on to my arms. I don't really know how long the grabbing and touching went on. I remember squirming to get free. I know a hand went up my private school skirt and there was laughter. Sinister, evil laughter. I heard a disconnected voice say, "Stop it!," not realizing it was my own. I can't remember everything that happened but there was my own, far away voice, yelling. "Knock it off!" But it was internal. The words would not, could not form vocally.

Then, the voice inside said, "RUN!" It took a second to shake the fog from my brain, to reconnect with my body, to what was happening with what I was thinking. Finally, I fought my way loose and ran until my lungs burned. Realizing they weren't chasing me, I slowed a bit but still double-timed it home.

I never told a soul what happened. A lifetime of messages that had been steeped from generation to generation taught me not to fight back. Those messages taught me that I was not valuable enough to speak up and have someone defend me. My sense of agency was nonexistent. I didn't believe in my value or that others would see value in me either. This was what I had inherited. It wrapped around my DNA, strangling who I was meant to be.

The next day at school, the boy I liked, the boy who stood by and did nothing, came to me and said his friends were only fooling and if I promised to never tell, he would be my boyfriend. I wanted the attention badly enough that I agreed. But I could not stand to look at him. Or at myself for that matter.

Even after we "broke up," I didn't see any point in telling anyone what had happened. Besides, they told me it was my own fault and what did I expect? It never occurred to me that they might be wrong. I had learned to take responsibility for everyone around me and if things didn't go well, it must be through some fault of my own.

The events of those days came simultaneously during lessons in our PE class about the importance of girls maintaining modesty and not being a temptation for boys. That solidified my belief that what happened was my fault. It likely emboldened the boy's accusations toward me as well.

They were very convincing in getting me to believe that given my problems at school and home, people would believe them over me anyway. After all, even teachers had made public comments that I was from a broken home and as such, had "a lot of problems." My belief that my value was less than theirs was affirmed. The boys convinced me that talking about what happened wouldn't bring about anything good for me. And the shame I felt over compromising with the boy I liked confirmed that idea.

While I decided not to *talk* about it, I did not know how to not *feel* anything about it. But I watched my mother and uncle rely on all variety of drink and drug to escape their reality. So, it felt perfectly reasonable to use substances as my escape route too. The only thing I could not figure out was what to do when the substances wore off and more shame set in. I did the only logical thing, and found more ways to numb, run and hide from my feelings.

Since there weren't any kids that I knew of my age engaging in the same sorts of behaviors, I leaned in more closely to my new, more "mature" friends who had access to all the supplies I needed to anesthetize myself from my life. It was the beginning of a deep dark spiral. One that, on more than one occasion, would almost cost me my life.

YOUR TURN: Reflect. Engage. Write.

Dear Friend, I'm curious to hear what patterns you recognize from one generation to the next at this point.

Some are not so obvious. Are you able to recognize how my environment growing up sent all sorts of messages about worth and contributed to confusion about who I was and who I was meant to be?

Does it make sense to you that I would engage in dangerous behaviors to escape the aftermath of my experiences?

Are there parts of my story and my behaviors that resonate with you and your story? Have you found yourself engaging in behaviors that are unsafe or unhealthy in the hopes they will numb you to the pain you've experienced? If so, journal about those behaviors and consider making a list of what they have cost you.

Please take a moment to journal your thoughts and consider sharing them with a trusted friend or counselor.

JUST LIKE THE BIG KIDS

I can't remember exactly how I met Kara and Mickey, but I think it was where all the tough kids hung out... the skating rink. Or more accurately, out back behind the joint... while smoking one. Quicker than you could say "do you want a hit?," they became my idols. These girls were just the right mix of mean, popular and sexy to give me a model for reinventing myself. I sort of became their "Barbie" that they could dress up in painted on jeans, painted on face, and set me up with the friends of the guys they liked. They were well-versed in the language of all things "boy." And they had access to all the drugs and alcohol a girl could want.

I saw these new friends as my way out. Out of school (they skipped *often*). Out of feeling bullied. (They were tough girls.) Out of my house. (They snuck me out to hang with them and their older male friends.)

These friends were such a big deal in my eyes. They were high schoolers, sophomores even! And while the kids in my eighth-grade class might've ruled the school yard, they were easily intimidated by these older, tougher girls who picked me up from the school yard *every* day. They also made it clear to my schoolmates that anyone who messed with me—guy or girl—messed with them. As unhealthy as it was, I felt protected and loved. Perhaps in their own dysfunctional way, that's what it was.

But their attention and protection came at a cost. Not that my new friends demanded or even requested anything specific from me. Rather, the cost was the natural consequence of hanging out with them and engaging in behaviors not meant for a 12-and-a-half-year-old. If there was any part of me that remained childlike, it wouldn't survive the new life I had embarked upon.

My home life became more and more constricting and I wanted to be with my new friends all the time. I avoided school like it was the plague since they rarely went to school themselves.

It felt good to feel seen by them and their friends. And to feel important. I was *really* enjoying the break from life that drugs and alcohol provided, not to mention the attention from the older guys that hung out with Kara and Mickey. It didn't seem to bother them that I was so young—not that any of them were asking my age. It helped (or didn't) that I looked at least four years older than my actual age (another family trait). And, as long as I did what they wanted, they kept me supplied with alcohol, drugs and more importantly, affection, which seemed like a fair trade to me.

The inexhaustible list of rules at home and school only intensified. What little conversation there had been between Judy and me before was consumed by her constant anger and punishment. Her tone rarely matched her words and her constant withholding of affection when she was angry caused my rebellious behaviors to rage. Eventually parenting me became too much to handle, and she completely disconnected—something I had done long before.

YOUR TURN: Reflect. Engage. Write.

My Dear Friend, this might be a good place to consider some of the behaviors that you have engaged in which allowed you to numb the pain of things you could not control in your world.

There are the obvious things like drugs and alcohol. But, as in the case of my story, there are other things like unhealthy and unsafe relationships.

As you take a pause to reflect on what you have read up to this point, are there any parts of my story that resonate with your own?

Can you see yourself (or others in your family) reflected in anyone who has been introduced in my story so far? If so, who and in what way(s)?

If so, this would be a good time to write down those thoughts.

CHAPTER 11

Deepening Distrust

MOVING OUT

In some ways, older friends filled a quasi-parenting role in my life. Though extremely dysfunctional, there was almost an element of nurturing to how they acted with me.

As experimental behaviors increased in their own lives, they did in my life as well. It wasn't long before I was smoking. So. Much. Pot. And "dating" the drug dealers so we could get it for free.

As much as it looked like I was having fun on the outside, I hated myself on the inside for not being able to say no to each temptation. But I feared a "no" meant they wouldn't want me around anymore. I feared that the "love and attention" they were showing me would be taken away. They were my lifeline. My escape. I also liked the way I didn't have to *feel* anything when I was high or drunk—all sunshine and roses. Oh, and I *really* liked their parents.

I looked for every and any excuse to be at their houses instead of my own. It was more peaceful there than with Mom Judy and Uncle Corky. No one seemed to be drunk. Or high. (Even if their kids were.) No one was violent or threatening. They spoke kindly to one another—no insults piercing anyone's heart.

Kara's and Mickey's parents were warm and welcoming. They were funny, cool and understanding. I wanted to be their kid too. The moms must have sensed this because both offered to let me call them "mom," which I happily accepted. I began to trust them more than I trusted my own parents. These moms showed me genuine concern. They had to have known something was amiss in my own home. What parent would allow their child to hang out with older kids like that and not ask any questions?

Granted, my friends got into trouble *occasionally*, but it was short lived and always seemed to be about what they had done rather than who they were. And I never got into trouble at their houses. I made sure I was as close to perfect as I could be in their eyes.

Still, I couldn't be with them *all* the time. So, I asked Ernie for more time with him in order to get away from Judy, but he said it wasn't possible because of his job. This might have been true, but I think the deeper reason was that he didn't feel equipped to handle me. He had his own story of abandonment and father wounds that remained unaddressed, so it made sense why he would struggle as a father himself. More time with him was not an option and I knew better than to ask Cathy, given her husband's opinion of me, not to mention the way he treated me. So, I was trapped in the chaos and it took a toll.

Eventually my health began to decline. Even as a small child, I constantly had issues with my stomach. Sometimes it would progress to headaches as well. I often had infections and generally felt ill. By the time I was nearing the end of eighth grade, nearly every facet of my world had

been impacted by the familial dysfunction and the dysfunction I was creating for myself. The impact of my homelife was manifesting in my physical body.

I regularly had migraines and debilitating stomach issues. These are known as Somatic experiences—the idea that trauma can manifest in physical symptoms. For children, headaches and stomach issues are among the most common. My menstrual periods also were horrendous, virtually from the first day of my first period. I had begun to experiment with boys before my body was ready for such things, and there is some research that would suggest that chronic stress along with early sexual behavior and even drug and alcohol use (all of which are hormone disruptors) may contribute to painful, heavy and unpredictable menstrual cycles.

Often the symptoms would leave me bed ridden and in pain, needing to stay home and rest. It was during one such period when, what was left of the bottom, fell out at home.

Judy had just come back from spending a night at the hospital due to yet another unfortunate reaction to a cocktail of pills and alcohol. She was barely functioning but went to work anyway. I had asked if I could stay home that morning, feeling extremely ill and exhausted. Judy flew into a rage and told me I needed to go to school. Which I did. It wasn't long into the day before I began to feel worse.

The principal called Judy to come get me, but she couldn't leave work. Corky couldn't be found. (Drunk at the bowling alley. Again.) So, the principal decided to send me home in a cab (they *actually* did things like that back in the day) and gave me instructions to immediately call Judy when I arrived and ask her to call the school to verify I was at home safely.

I assumed the school informed Judy that they were sending me home in a cab, but they didn't. When I obediently called her at work, I no sooner

got the words "I'm home and I'm going to bed" out of my mouth when she exploded.

"I've had *enough* of your shit! I can't *deal* with you anymore. *I'm putting you in a home*!" Those were the words she *said*. But, the words I *heard* were more along the lines of *"I don't want you anymore and I can't deal with your shit so I'm sending you somewhere else so they can deal with you."*

I panicked. My heart raced. My brain was screaming, *"you've got to get out of here before she puts you in a home!"* And that was the first (but not the last) time I ran away.

After frantic, failed attempts to get in touch with Ernie, I packed a small suitcase and headed for my older friend Mickey's house. Her mom defended me and called her husband.

I overheard her on the phone with him, "If her mother says she's really going to send her to a home, we have to take her in. You know what happens in *those* places?" I didn't know what happened at "those places" but I was grateful for people who would fight to keep it from happening to me.

Mickey's mom asked me for my Dad's phone number, and I was afraid to give it to her because I had no idea what he would do. Maybe he would agree with Judy. *"Maybe he should,"* I thought. *"Maybe I really am too much to handle."*

Mickey's mom promised she wouldn't let anything bad happen to me, so I gave her the number.

I didn't hear their conversation, but she told me Ernie was coming to pick me up and that if things didn't work out, I should call her right away

and she would come get me. Her words and actions made me feel less alone. And I was grateful—but still afraid.

When Ernie picked me up, we drove the few short blocks to Judy's house. I realize it might sound weird that I don't call it "my house," but the truth is, I don't really remember anywhere I lived in my childhood truly feeling like home. That says more about my internal state during childhood than it does about the brick and mortar that surrounded me.

When we arrived, he told me not to say anything at first and suggested I go to my room, close the door and quietly listen to music. I happily complied, save for pressing the side of my head to the door so I could hear what they were saying in the event I needed to make a quick run-for-it back to Mickey's.

Ernie got straight to the point with Judy. "Have you calmed down yet?"

"I have," she replied in her iciest tone, reserved mostly for him, and me when I was headed for *really* big trouble.

"But I meant what I said. I'm not dealing with her anymore. Either she lives with you or she goes to a home. I'm done."

Those words transported me back to when I was a small child, walking around watching the scowls and hearing the tsks of my family. Wondering what I had done wrong and how I could fix it. Praying someone would tell me what to do. Hoping that someone would make it all right. Desperately needing someone to make *me* all right.

Something broke in me that night. It wasn't the first incident of breaking, but it was an important one. If there was any thread of connection between Judy and me remaining, it was severed with this final betrayal of trust. I knew that I would need to let go of any part of me that still held out hope for Judy to be the mother I needed, the mother I so desperately

wanted. Once again, I was reminded that my only hope of being safe was to be an adult and take care of myself.

But one cannot simply "will themselves" into being developmentally ready for responsibility like that. No matter how dire the circumstances or how badly I wanted it. Like it or not, I was still technically dependent, which meant I would need to depend on someone to help me. And it looked like Ernie was it.

When he entered my room, I was sitting crisscross on my rainbow latch hook rug that took forever to make.

"Come on, Kiddo," he sighed. "Grab a few things and we'll come back for the rest. You're coming to stay with me."

I can't remember what all I grabbed. I'm sure I grabbed my makeup. And I'm sure I grabbed my favorite clothes. But I think I left the latch hook rug, too busy wondering what I would need to do to keep him from wanting to get rid of me too.

A FINAL BLOW TO INNOCENCE

Trigger Warning: Some of the material in this chapter may be difficult to read, particularly if you've had any trauma or abuse of a sexual nature in your past. Feel free to skip this chapter or at a minimum, proceed with caution. And promise both of us (that's yourself and me) that you will stop reading if it becomes too triggering or painful.

Moving in with Ernie was lightning fast. One minute I was living with Judy and Corky within walking distance of school. The next I was in a new home, new neighborhood and new routine. The one-bedroom, shotgun apartment that he maintained was insufficient for the two of us

long term. So, he purchased a home within walking distance of school *and* Judy.

The skills I had acquired out of necessity when living with Judy came in handy when living with Ernie. I could cook, but just simple dishes. At least they were edible. I could also clean and do laundry, skills Ernie was pleased with. My help in those areas seemed to reduce the stress of having me there.

I did *a lot* of cooking and cleaning and laundry. But I did not do a lot of interacting with Ernie. I often felt like a burden and my desire to connect with him felt like a source of pain and frustration. I longed to be taken care of, yet had an inherent inability to trust anyone to do the job. I still needed the love and affection that every child needs, but I don't know that I would have been capable of receiving it even if it was offered. Although he was incapable of parenting me the way I needed, I want to make it clear that out of everyone, I believe he tried the hardest.

As hard as he tried, most of the time Ernie was exhausted from working hard and being a single dad. He didn't put up much of an argument when my older friends asked me to come over. I continued to seek out relationships with older individuals who could fill the role of parent in one form or another. From that point on, the friends got older and the guys got a little more dangerous. I quickly graduated to "friends" in their twenties.

Ernie never seemed to mind when I spent time with them or when I asked to spend the night with friends either. My friend Kara's father, Mr. D, seemed to take a special interest in me and my challenges at home. He would often tell Ernie not to worry about picking me up and usually offered for me to stay for dinner, telling my dad that he would let his daughter use the car to drive me home afterwards. It was nice to feel as though someone was taking an interest.

One particular evening Ernie had to work late, and my friend's father offered once again for me to stay for dinner and get a ride home with them afterwards. When the time came to drive me home, Mr. D reminded Kara that she was technically still grounded, so not only was she restricted from using the car, but she wasn't allowed to accompany us on the drive back to my house. As Kara protested further, he reminded her she was lucky he even allowed me to come and hang out at all. She rolled her eyes so hard I could almost hear them hitting her eyelids. "Sorry." She said, shrugging her shoulders. "It's OK," I smiled and shrugged back, "see you tomorrow."

On the way home, Mr. D struck up the normal conversation. "Did you girls have fun tonight?" A typical question, which was a less than veiled attempt at extracting intel on what we might be plotting for the weekend.

"Yeah," I said, "it was fun. And thanks for dinner." It was awkward being with him by myself and I was anxious to get home.

"Hey!" he said with enthusiasm, "Has your dad taught you how to drive yet?"

"No," I said with a laugh, "I don't think he believes I'm ready for that."

"Well, you're going to be old enough for a permit before you know it! So, you should learn," he said firmly.

"OK, if you think so." I had no idea where he was going with all of that and I didn't want to argue with him, so I just shrugged and agreed. Besides, I kind of liked the idea that he thought I was ready to learn how to drive.

"Slide on over here," he chuckled, extending his arm to his side to make way for me to sit close enough to him to get the driver's point of view. "You steer and I'll work the pedals." He motioned for me to take the

wheel. He showed me how to keep the car steady and to make sure my grip was firm on the wheel, ten-and-two and all that jazz. "And no matter what," he warned, *"never* take your eyes off the road."

After a few minutes I started to get the hang of it. He told me I had complete control of the car but no matter what, not to take my eyes off the road or let go of the wheel because we might crash.

"I'm going to speed up so you can see how it feels to control the car. Remember, *you're* in control. Don't let go of the wheel and don't take your eyes off the road."

"Geez," I thought to myself. *"I get it!"*

As he accelerated, I felt a little uneasy and told him I was ready to give him back the wheel, but Mr. D reassured me that he was right there, and if anything happened, he would be able to take control.

As I relaxed a bit more, he put his arm around my shoulders to let me get even closer to the driver's point of view. He asked me if I felt more in control from that vantage point. I felt unsure but didn't want to disappoint him, so I told him I did. I no sooner said that when his hand slipped below my arm and in between my legs. My head snapped in his direction and he took my face and pointed it back to the road.

"Don't look away or we'll crash," he whispered in my ear.

I was frozen. My stomach rolled.

"Now, doesn't that feel nice?" The tone in his voice indicated he didn't really want an answer.

I couldn't speak and I couldn't move. I didn't know what to do. My mind was screaming at me to do something, but I couldn't. I had no words.

Incapable of action. It all felt familiar yet different. I momentarily flashed back to that fateful walk home with the boys from school. But this felt darker, and more confusing.

Mr. D wasn't physically violent, but his grip on me was vice-like. He was firm, making sure I knew he was in control, but tried to make his voice sound soft and coaxing. To me it sounded sinister, as my body and mind became a dark mix of confusion. He continued his assault as panic mixed with other, troubling sensations. My body seemed to betray me as I felt my mind attempt to detach.

Abruptly, he took the wheel with one hand and grabbed my hand with the other, pressing it firmly against his crotch. I thought for sure I was going to throw up. Finally, he lightened his grip, and I was able to wrestle my hand away and slide as far away from him as I could without exiting a moving vehicle. I pressed my face against the cold window glass and squeezed my eyes shut tight, attempting to will myself out of the car in my mind.

He quickly finished himself to the point of release, then told me I should never say anything to my dad because I would be in big trouble and he would destroy my relationship with Kara.

I didn't know what to do, but any fleeting thoughts of telling my father left my head immediately when we got out of the car and my friend's dad began talking with my father about football and how difficult it must be to be a single dad. I all but ran into the house, as Mr. D shouted, "thanks for the talk on the way home, honey. See you soon."

I wanted to throw up. I raced up the steps and into the house, peering at the two of them through the sheers and listening through the crack in the open window, willing him to leave. I wished my dad could just *know,* without me having to say anything.

Mr. D seemed to look right through the window and into my soul, directing a dark smirk toward the house over Ernie's shoulder, sending a chill up my spine. I was flooded with shame.

"If you ever need any help with Gina, just give me a call. It's no trouble at all." I heard him offer as he got into the car. He emphasized to my father what good friends his daughter and I were and how I was always welcome in their home.

When my father came walking towards the house with a smile on his face, I beelined for my room. I shut the door, grunting a response to him when he asked if I had a good time. I couldn't wait until he settled in for his evening distraction in front of the TV so I could pop open my window and smoke a joint. Or three. I wondered if I could sneak a couple of Ernie's beers without him noticing, then decided it was worth the risk of getting caught. I snatched three from the fridge and downed them in rapid succession, anxious for the familiar high of the drugs and alcohol, longing for them to take me away from all I had experienced that evening.

I never told my father what happened that night. For many years, I never told anyone.

Mr. D would attempt the same behavior with me a few more times in different scenarios before it finally sunk in that I could never be alone with him—not even when other people were in his home. I would need to walk myself home in the dark, through uncertain streets and lie to my father about how I got there in order to be safe. I hated myself for wishing that it could be different with Mr. D, and for giving him more than one chance to harm me.

Sadly, that night wouldn't be the only encounter that left me confused about the relationship between sex and my worth. Those beliefs would be further compromised by an uncle who I believed wanted to be a

father figure to me. My experience with him was a repeat of what happened with Mr. D (though not in a moving vehicle). The unaddressed aftermath of these traumatic experiences, and those earlier in life, ushered in so much shame and confusion about my worth. Understandably, between the ages of 13 and 25, I ended up in sexually and emotionally abusive relationships with boyfriends much older than me.

After my encounters with Mr. D, I just wanted to do whatever it took to forget. I didn't want to think or feel anything. I just wanted to disappear. Since I couldn't figure out how to literally do that, I did the next best thing and began taking drugs and/or drinking like it was my job, an everyday occurrence.

I was 13 years old.

I walked around like I hated everyone. But most of all, I hated myself. While Ernie had no idea what I had been through or what I was doing, he knew I was getting worse. Worse in my behaviors, my attitude, lying—all of it. The spiral was palpable.

I would still see Judy from time to time, but mostly, I stayed away from her. While I professed deep disdain towards her, I was really just a wounded little girl who wished her mom wanted her around more.

Unable to admit that truth, I continued to keep up my tough-girl front. I skipped school more than I attended, often running around Judy's neighborhood with my friends, intentionally tempting fate.

YOUR TURN: Reflect. Engage. Write.

Dear Friend, it might have been difficult to hear this portion of the story. While I have worked through these events in therapy; admittedly, it's still difficult to write them here, for all to read. But it's important that I share my experiences using my out loud voice. Not just for myself, but for others who have yet to tell their stories, to encourage them. And to encourage you, if this is a part of your past.

There are many people with sexual abuse (and abuses of all kinds, for that matter) in their childhood who continue to blame themselves and feel somehow complicit in what happened because they continued to be around their abuser, particularly if the predator offered something that felt like love and nurturing that their victim wasn't getting from their caregiver(s).

Aside from the more violent and forceful violations of victims, there are some who have experienced abuse that wasn't necessary *physically* violent, even if it was sexual in nature. But the results and emotional scars are traumatic, nonetheless. Bodily sensations mixed with the knowledge that what is happening is wrong can further complicate a victim's internal state of blame. This can make it confusing to label experiences as abuse, and feelings of connection to the abuser can cause debilitating shame and internal blame.

Lastly, there are instances where abuse is a family legacy. It isn't talked about, but rather, denied and/or held as a family secret. Or, perhaps it's not taken seriously because the abuser is regarded as "a good person," so in the eyes of friends and family, that individual couldn't *possibly* be abusive.

But here's the thing: abusers don't abuse everyone they meet. And there is a reason why they are called "predators."

If any of this resonates with your story, let me say this clearly: *no matter what happened, no matter what you did or didn't do, it was never*

> *your fault. Not in even the smallest sense of the word.* Even if you continued to allow yourself to be around your abuser.
>
> That desire for acceptance? That need for love and connection that drove you to risk being around that person? It stems from our natural desire for acceptance and connection. It is wired into us, imperative to our survival. It would stand to reason you would want that. The fact that your desire for these good and natural things was exploited and distorted by someone isn't your fault.
>
> Please, Precious Soul, do not blame yourself for what happened to you. And if you never have before, please tell your story to a trusted someone today. Begin to heal. Get the help you deserve. God doesn't intend for you to carry the weight of someone else's offenses. Put. It. Down.

FAILED ATTEMPT TO GET HELP

One day when I was skipping school, my friends and I came down the hill near Judy's house and I noticed her car was there.

"We should stop by," I said sarcastically. "She doesn't care what I do." But we were high, and while my rebellious nature wanted to flaunt that in front of her, my friends were less courageous, so we went on about our day instead.

Later that night, Ernie got a call from Corky, asking us to come over to the house he still shared with Judy. Ernie waited until the very last minute when we were turning on her street to tell me that Judy had died at some point earlier that morning. I overheard the paramedics found 23 active prescriptions in the cabinet where she kept her meds—many in my grandmother Julie's name, who had died years before.

I remember thinking to myself, *"if I had stopped by, could I have saved her?"* The thought haunted me; what could have been. My adoptive mother died with so many things left unresolved and unhealed between us, just like my biological mother Cathy had experienced with her own mother, Marie. I hated Judy for dying. It felt like the ultimate act of giving up on me. My resentment was so strong, fighting against my ability to grieve. And still, the spiral deepened.

With so much out of control in my life, magnified by Judy's death, Ernie took a friend's advice and found us a counselor. We became close with her and eventually I ended up spending a fair amount of time with her and her husband at their home. Her intervention in my life was initially a welcome distraction. She had no children of her own and seemed to see potential in me that others didn't. Slowly, I dipped my toe in the waters of trusting her. I appreciated the attention she gave and felt like I had someone in my corner for the first time in a long time. The last night I would spend time in her home was a sleepover during one of my terrible menstrual periods.

I was complaining to her that my lower back hurt and she offered to give me a massage. It began to border on inappropriate, so I made up an excuse that I was feeling sick to my stomach. That part was actually true. I just didn't tell her it was because of the way she was touching me. I said that I wanted to go to sleep. I didn't want to make her mad and I didn't want to lose her attention and affection. I just didn't want it in *that* way. But with this new violation, the memory of the old ones came back.

Here was yet another adult in my life who couldn't be trusted. Or maybe there was just something wrong with *me*. I came to the conclusion that my worth must be based purely on what I had to offer physically. After all, it couldn't be that there was something wrong with *every* adult who wasn't my parent, right?

It must be me.

That was the last time I spent the night at the counselor's house. After that, I began to rebel against her advice in counseling. I told Ernie we didn't need her anymore. I think part of him felt conflicted. But a bigger part of him felt relieved.

Eventually, like a Jenga game where each block pulled from the structure shifts and compromises its foundation, my relationship with Ernie became a shaky place. My unraveling from there was quick and deeply plagued with more substance abuse, dangerous and abusive relationships and even abortion. From there, for a near decade and a half, my life was a blur.

Ernie and I became estranged from one another, although over the years there were times when I would reach out to see if we could cobble together some semblance of a relationship. All of that came to a screeching halt when after one of our falling outs, he said, "I don't know, Gina. I think it would just be easier for me if I pretended like I didn't have a daughter anymore."

I didn't know what to say. I was 22, but the feeling took me back to when Judy threatened to put me in a home. I could feel the little girl in me wanting to rise up, beg Ernie to change his mind. Inside, I was hoping he would tell me what I could do to change his mind. But the tough girl in me wouldn't let her take the risk of asking. Instead I lashed out in the childish hopes of hurting him the way he had just hurt me. I'll never know if my cutting response (one I don't fully remember) hit its mark because I never spoke to him again.

Based on what I know of Ernie's childhood (abandonment and poverty), he had his own unresolved issues when he became my father. Having kept his past and how he felt about it a secret from others (and from himself), I imagine engaging in therapy with and for me was a struggle for him. I say that because being in therapy for yourself or with family requires a certain introspection. If you can't come to grips with some

of your own emotions and experiences, it will be difficult to meet your own kids in whatever they are going through. If I look back, knowing what I know now, I can only imagine how difficult that whole situation must've been for him, trying to help me navigate emotional waters he refused to enter himself. Once again, it emphasizes the importance of working through our story in order to be the healthiest we can be to help to our kids. No matter what they go through.

CHAPTER 12 A Science Break

MISSING TIME AND THE BODY'S RESPONSE

It's probably not surprising that much of my childhood is a blur to me. As I mentioned in the very beginning of this book, in cases of chronic trauma and neglect, pervasive chaos and instability, this occurrence of "missing time" is actually quite common. It took a while for me to let go of the shame that came with my experience of it. People would ask me about my childhood or my life, and I would struggle to make sense of the story I wanted to share. My narrative lacked cohesiveness. Memories were spotty. They still are. Sometimes I get it out of order. Sometimes I need to go back and correct myself. Other times a new piece of information surfaces and helps me put things into perspective. For some of my memory to come back, I had to heal from the shame and fear before my brain would allow the information to resurface. But the parts I *do* know? I *really* know.

You might struggle with some of the same issues, so I want you to know that just because some parts are missing, that doesn't mean you don't *really* know the parts that you *can* remember, regardless of its

cohesiveness. It's important for me to tell you that, because as a child I was often told that what I experienced wasn't *really* real. Other times, I was threatened and told not to retell something I heard, saw, or something that happened to me.

I spent a lot of time trying to push down memories and tell myself that what happened didn't really happen. Maybe you've had similar experiences and it's brought you shame, pain or frustration. Maybe, like me, it's brought you all three. If that's the case, although we cannot physically be together at this moment, please hear me when I say, "I see you. I'm with you. And you are *not* crazy." What you've experienced makes sense to me and I believe you. By the way, it makes sense from a clinical perspective, too.

When a person lives in a state of heightened chaos or pervasive trauma and/or neglect, particularly for extended periods of time, a portion of the brain, called the amygdala, gets stuck in the "on" position. Typically, the amygdala signals us that danger is present and instructs us on how to protect ourselves by either fight, flight or freeze. However, when we live in a state of constant danger, the amygdala goes into overdrive. Consequently, the part(s) of the brain that can tell us all is well and that we are safe is silenced; taken off-line, if you will. The stress hormone cortisol rules the day and floods the brain which can have significant negative impact not only on the brain, but on the body as a whole.

One important area of the brain that is negatively impacted as a result of this overflow of cortisol is the hippocampus. The hippocampus is responsible for helping us manage our memories and develop our self-narrative (the story we tell ourselves and others about who we are).

Our hippocampus can sort of atrophy, making it difficult to form a cohesive narrative, in part because trauma isn't readily "understandable" to our brain. We don't really have a true context for trauma. Our brain knows trauma is something that isn't *supposed* to happen. This helps to

explain our responses/reactions to trauma when it occurs or when we recall it.

Additionally, behaviors we engage in to attempt to anesthetize our experiences, like the drinking and substance abuse I engaged in, as well as toxic relationships, are terribly corrosive. Not to mention, alcohol and drug abuse delays the development of an adolescent brain, including the hippocampal regions, even when there hasn't been other trauma. (Most of us can think of at least one person we know who began using substances at a young age and consequently, they seem sort of stuck at that age. They might be an adult chronologically, but relationally, emotionally and behaviorally, they're like an adolescent.)

The need to anesthetize can also play out in other ways, like addiction to dangerous situations. This was true for me. I had little regard for my own physical safety, let alone emotional safety. I went where the wind blew me, as long as it allowed me to engage in behaviors to disconnect from the pain inside. Regardless of the cost. Sometimes to myself. Sometime to others.

SCIENCE MEETS SCRIPTURE: TRANSGENERATIONAL EPIGENETIC INHERITANCE

I was developmentally ill-equipped to handle most of the freedoms and experiences I had in my childhood and teen years. It was deeply unhealthy for me to have such experiences at such a critical developmental stage of life. In early adolescence, what we're exposed to impacts us deeply. This is the part of life where we begin to look at what it means to be us. We try on different hats. Make decisions about friend groups. We start to solidify language about ourselves that we will take on as our identity. While this begins and continues throughout our young lives, adolescence is the time when beliefs about ourselves and others become solidified into the stories by which we live.

Although I had older friends who were bad influences on me at times, the truth is that even before these friends came into my life, I had developed strong beliefs about myself and others which guided me to the path I walked. These were beliefs passed down through the generations. I now see the destructive narrative I adopted based on my life experiences and the agreements I had made with myself about who I was, my value and the trustworthiness of others and even of God. All of those "agreements" were rooted in shame. And if shame is part of your foundation, it is likely to determine your ceiling, with little to no clearance to hold your head up high. Shame can be a legacy of its own. And there is science to prove it.

If shame is part of your foundation, it is likely to determine your ceiling, with little to no clearance to hold your head up high. Shame can be a legacy of its own. And there is science to prove it.

Transgenerational Epigenetic Inheritance is a science-y term that means the transmission of information from one generation of an organism to the next (i.e., parent–child transmission) that affects the traits of offspring without alteration of the primary structure of DNA—in other words, *epigenetically* rather that *genetically*. Still too science-y?

Try this:

Transgenerational Epigenetic Inheritance tells us what we pass down to the next generation is more than just our genes. It's the influences that express or suppress their expression as well. Research shows that what we are exposed to in our life changes and molds our "make-up." We can then pass down the resulting traits to the next generation. And the next. Without the knowledge of what the generations before us experienced, we run the risk of those patterns expressing themselves in our lives and feeling as though we have no control over it. We accept it as "just how it is," never questioning if it could possibly be different.

When we grow up in an unhealthy environment where dysfunctional beliefs, habits and relationships are modeled, we often adopt those same habits into our own way of doing life as adults. We aren't necessarily inheriting a "gene" for dysfunction. But we have, in a way, inherited the *epigenetics* for the dysfunction, the tendency toward or away from it.

But here's where I believe Scripture truly informs Science. We aren't really wired to live dysfunctional lives. We're wired for healthy love and connection. Healthy connections are key for our wellbeing emotionally, physically, mentally and spiritually. This is our truest inherent design. We don't have to learn how to love or learn to desire connection. It's just in us.

On the other hand, we *do* learn to fear certain things and to become disconnected. And while our experiences in life might give us cause to operate out of fear and disconnection, it isn't part of our original design. But hang on. Because here's where the hope is...

> If we learned these behaviors as a result of our experiences, then it stands to reason we can unlearn those same behaviors and then replace them with new experiences and new ways of thinking. This empowers us to transform ourselves, to be molded more in line with how we are designed: to love, to be loved and to be connected.

Scripture gives us many insights into what that transformation can look like and how we might get there. And research as well suggests that transformation is possible and is influenced by our choices, behavior and environment.

We could even go so far as to say that some genes can be turned on or off at certain stages in our lives, depending on the behaviors we engage in and environments we are exposed to. Here's an example. Say that a

grandparent was an alcoholic, but you never knew. Your parents knew it though, and consequently never used alcohol to manage emotions, deal with life or even in social settings. As a result of your parents' choices, you never saw alcohol abused or really used at all. Fast forward to adolescence and you're at a party where emotions are running high and peer pressure is intense enough to crack concrete.

Not wanting to be on the receiving end of ridicule, you decide to drink. And drink. And drink. Given the stage of life, the emotional conditions under which you use alcohol (or any mood/mind altering drug, for that matter), you run the risk of "turning on" the genes that predispose you to alcoholism from a heredity perspective.

Fast forward a few years and without intervention, the problem intensifies. Or worsens. Or cross-pollinates into other forms of addiction. You may even wonder how you got there because you never saw anyone in your family struggle with addiction. No one had ever mentioned it to you. You never saw your parent(s) abuse alcohol or any other substance. What you don't realize (and perhaps neither do they) is that their manifestation of addiction may have played out in other ways. Workaholic. Gym-a-holic. Perfectionist. While those behaviors are much more acceptable in our society, and even celebrated in some circles, they are manifestations of that same addictive pattern that took a more destructive route in your life.

Perhaps addiction didn't manifest itself at all in your parent's lives. Maybe knowing they were predisposed to it and abstaining from substances was a decision they made as a result of choosing to be healthy emotionally, physically and mentally. Perhaps they even sought help dealing with what growing up in an alcoholic household was like. They worked through it so your exposure to the consequences of grandpa's alcoholism was minimal or non-existent. Maybe all that work they did personally made them believe grandpa's addiction was something you never needed to know about. But contrary to the popular saying, sometimes the things we don't know *can* hurt us.

If you remember, as we walked through the generations before me, it was emotional strife and struggle and a crisis of identity that seemed to lead my grandmother into using prescription drugs and alcohol. With that, her behaviors point to an addiction to relationships as well, working herself into one relationship or the next to find her value.

The emotional wounds seemed to pass on to my mother, heightened first by the loss of her father's presence in her life, and then her mother's. Eventually the emotional wounds played out in her life through excessive use of alcohol, promiscuity and a deep uncertainty in her sense of self and her worth. These were then passed on to me.

While each of us had our own set of circumstances that would make healthfulness nearly impossible without some interventions, it is undeniable that what each generation endured before it significantly contributed to the dysfunction of the generations after them. For many years the hallmark of legacy in my family was soul-suffocating shame. This kind of shame can be the result of any number of emotional wounds, sometimes physical ones as well. It forms in those places where events and circumstances have caused you to believe there is something fundamentally wrong with *who* you are. At your core. It taints all you believe; all you do and all that you are.

And this is another reason why it's so important to uncover what has contributed to our lives from the generations before us. When we realize some of our most destructive behaviors and ways of thinking didn't originate with us, we find another level of freedom to release them, because they weren't really ours to begin with. They were something we unknowingly adopted to adapt in our environment. Discovering this helps us to think differently about what we believe and consequently how we behave.

GIVEN UP TWICE–REVISITED

Remember at the beginning of the book when I told you that my biological mother, Cathy, had given me up for adoption twice? Well, if you don't mind taking a little walk backward with me, I think we should take a deeper look at why this is such an important event.

The fallout I experienced from my adoption events and the disruption in bonding to caregivers that it created are called *attachment wounds*. In therapy, identifying experiences like these is extremely helpful. Having this information can help make sense of certain challenges in our relationships, perception of self, the ability to trust and bond with people, and even struggles in a relationship with God.

The problem was that I didn't know any of this when I entered therapy. So, while I had the privilege of working with wonderful therapists who truly understood the importance of taking a holistic approach to helping me, this essential portion of my story remained hidden from them. It took a long time and some assuming on both my part and the part of my therapists to incorporate attachment work into my therapy. But it didn't really take root for a while. I was unable to recognize the relevance of that work until much later in my journey.

The discovery of this new(er) information and its implications made me angry. And just for a moment, I felt the sting of abandonment and insecurity once again. I also felt a sense of betrayal. If I had known the truth about my adoption, and even about the things my biological mother had endured in her own life, I could have given that information to my highly qualified therapists and we could've made a plan of escape from my wilderness much quicker. And that's not to mention how helpful some of the generational information could have been—information about patterns of dysfunction, addiction, betrayal, abandonment, and the like.

It could've been like a map from point A to point B. That doesn't mean the road would have been a straight and bump-free ride. It just means we might have done a better job of anticipating the potholes and been able to fill at least some of them in along the way.

Fortunately, working through the discovery of this information hasn't been as slow as it once might have been. The lenses through which I see myself and my biological mother have changed color over the years. My vision has cleared. And it's been bittersweet, with grief and pain—but with grace and mercy and forgiveness as well.

Learning of the chaos that surrounded me as an infant and toddler has provided me with a deeper sense of self-compassion and a deeper understanding of why finding healthy relationships and being healthy myself was such a difficult journey.

For many years (even after I entered therapy) I would often ask myself why the journey was so difficult. Why couldn't I just get it together? What was my deal with not being able to trust people? Why did I always need to be in control or manipulate to ensure that terrible, awful things wouldn't happen? Why did I think the slightest delay in communication with someone I loved or an unmet request meant the person didn't love me or was going to leave? And why did I seem to constantly choose emotionally unavailable, and even abusive relationships? Why did I have such a fragile sense of self and why did I constantly feel the need to reinvent myself to please the people around me?

Discovering the attachment wounds of my past allowed me to understand that my earliest life experiences with parents and grandparents left a mark. Nurture affects nature. We are shaped by our experiences. And until we understand what has shaped us and how we can go about creating new, corrective experiences to mold us into who we are created to be, we will struggle from the pain of our wounds, whether they're from attachment, abuse or pervasive exposure to unhealthy choices of our caregivers.

In other words, to get to where we want to go, we must first understand from where it is we have come and what got us there. We may not need to recall every minute detail, but we do need to recognize the impact our experiences have had on us, and the maladaptive behaviors we've developed as a result.

For me (and others you will briefly read about in Part Eight), understanding came from discovering information about more than just our parents, but learning about the generations before as well.

Here's a light-hearted allegory to draw a picture of what I mean. The original story is from motivational guru Zig Ziglar. I've heard it often over the years with slight variations here and there, but about a decade ago, I began to take some poetic license with it. The tale that follows is the result.

Once upon a time there was a mom who made the most incredible Easter feasts. Each year she enjoyed creating unique, mouth-watering dishes to the delight of her family.

In time, she had a daughter who, as she grew, became more and more interested in making the Easter feasts. In particular, she wanted to learn how to make the star of the show, the Easter ham.

Each year the ham was served with nary the slightest variation, adorned in pineapple slices, cherry halves and deep, black cloves.

And each year… It. Was. Glorious.

Year after year, the young girl watched as her mother strategically and carefully recreated this delicacy. Especially how mom would masterfully adorn it with garnish and with the precision of a skilled surgeon, she would slice the ends off the ham and place it gingerly into the heavy black and white speckled pan, before sliding its girth into the oven.

Finally, the glorious Easter came when it was Daughter's turn to prepare the Easter feast! She closed her eyes and recalled just how mom had done it all the years before. Her copy of the ham was sheer perfection, down to every last cherry and clove. She trimmed off the ends evenly and baked accordingly. It turned out fabulous!

Mother was so proud.

Many Easters flew by (as Easters often do). Daughter became a wife and mother herself. Before long, the time came to pass the torch onto her own daughter. A tradition now three generations deep.

And as on countless Easters before, now the third generation-master-chef set about preparing the ham, duplicating it to pure perfection, as mother and grandmother looked on.

Then, one year… just as everything was going to plan, something changed.

And mother noticed immediately.

"Sweetheart, you forgot to cut the ends off the ham." She said, sounding a bit miffed that daughter would omit such an important step.

"Oh, well, I was thinking it might be better if I left them on," her daughter replied, as she placed the ham in her new, shiny red baking pan.

"Well," mom replied with a hint of defensiveness, "your grandmother always cut the ends off, and I have always cut the ends off. Up until now, even you cut the ends off. And every year the ham has turned out delicious! I don't know why you would want to change it."

While daughter didn't want to argue, especially on a holiday, she was certain her way of cooking would turn out better. So, she gently pressed in a little deeper.

"Mom, why do we need to cut off the ends? How does that make it better?" she asked.

Slightly exasperated, Mother replied, "Because…" she stopped cold, a very puzzled look spreading across her face, then in frustration said, "well, I'll let Grandma tell you why."

"What's wrong?" Grandma could feel the tension in the room as she entered.

"Mom, will you please come in here and tell your granddaughter why we cut the ends off the ham. She wants to cook it with the ends on. Can you imagine? She's going to ruin the whole thing!"

Grandmother looked at the ham in the pan and furrowed her brow; a long pause passing. Then a relaxed, but somewhat sad, smile crept across her face.

"Oh, sweetheart, let her cook it the way she wants. The pan I used all those years was my mother's and I didn't want to get a new one. I only cut the ends off because the ham wouldn't fit into the pan."

The. Ham. Wouldn't. Fit. In. The. Damn. Pan.

All it took was a simple question, *two generations in the making,* to reveal a pattern so implicit, yet so pervasive that it was believed to be the only way to "cook the ham."

A little discussion revealed that not only was there more than one way to cook the ham, there was, in fact a better way that prevented the unnecessary trimming. Perhaps grandmother could've owned the fact that her pan was too small, that she didn't want to give up her mother's pan or that they didn't have enough money to buy a new, bigger one.

Maybe she could've taught her daughter that there was a different, even better way. When she saw that her granddaughter's pan was indeed big enough to accommodate the larger ham, she could've stopped her from cutting off the ends of the ham. But she didn't. Why? Perhaps the old and unnecessary way of doing things had become so deeply ingrained it simply didn't occur to her there could be a better way.

How many other areas of life and behavior had been handed down the same way? And how many more questions would granddaughter know to ask to affect change without being given the raw data to know what kind of questions needed asking? Or worse, how many behaviors would she repeat, how many beliefs would she adopt as her own, never realizing there is a different, or better way? How many consequences that go way beyond a dry ham would she experience? How many did she run the risk of passing on to generations after her?

It took three generations to discover that ham, in fact, is better with the ends on. That you can buy a bigger pan. And apparently, you don't need the permission of the generations before to do so. And *that,* is an allegory for my life.

Without understanding fully where many of the seemingly intrinsic and reflexive behaviors originated, I acted upon assumptions about myself and the world around me that weren't true. But I had to find the pieces of my story, and the stories of those before me, that evaded me before I could figure out that I didn't need to "cut the ends off the ham." After all, you don't know what you don't know until you know it. Then, when you know, you must do something with it. Because knowledge is only power when it's combined with action.

Knowledge is only power when it's combined with action.

YOUR TURN: Reflect. Engage. Write.

Take a moment and journal whatever came to mind as you read through this chapter, including the story about the ham. Perhaps this stirred some thoughts about your own family. Even about some of your family traditions or of things done just because it's always been done this way or that way.

In terms of what you read about attachment wounds, how do you relate to this section?

Journal any other stories you might know from your own life or Scripture that speak to Transgenerational Epigenetic Inheritance as you now understand it.

CHAPTER 13

Adulthood

TOO MANY JAGGED LITTLE PILLS

In my teens and young adult years, I kept running at a frenetic pace, on a quest for belonging. And I tried living in *a lot* of places, but a geographical cure held no relief for what ailed me. If I lived in Missouri, California, Illinois or on the moon, nothing seemed to bring me the love and care I so desperately needed. Those in whom I hoped and foolishly believed could do the job wasn't limited to those we've already discussed. In fact, my choices didn't improve much with age. Beyond a drug dealer, there were the rich and famous, prominent businessmen, a DEA agent (since the drug dealer didn't work out, I thought I'd go the opposite direction) and a couple rock stars.

My adventures took me many places and offered many experiences. One tiny perk that comes from living a chaotic and dangerous lifestyle is that you have no fear in saying "yes" to what many might find terrifying or at the very least, incredibly intimidating. What you fear is when the bright lights fade, the loud music ends and you come down from the high of your latest drug, drink or relationship, you're left with yourself

and the emptiness that you feel. And because that emptiness is so suffocating, you look for the next sensational thing, one more outrageous than the next, to keep the emptiness at bay.

Through my teens and early 20's, (most of those years spent in a drug and alcohol induced haze), I experienced the most incredible of extremes, following in my biological mom's "wild" footsteps, and perhaps even taking it up a notch. To onlookers, my highs might have been considered impressively high (no pun intended). But my lows were subterranean. While I had some brushes with fame, hobnobbing with "hair band" royalty, I was drawn in by the counterfeit sense of worth from their performance-based attention and fickle fans. I've even performed on stage in front of thousands, moving from place to place, meeting countless people, craving any sliver of acceptance those shallow connections offered.

But on the flip side, I've been completely homeless, with nowhere to go and no one to care.

I've dined in some of the fanciest restaurants and visited some amazing sights around the country and even the world. But I also know what it's like to write bad checks to cover groceries or medication.

When I modeled, and I use that term loosely (it was short-lived and a *horrible* choice for someone with zero self-worth or boundaries), I landed several "legitimate" gigs, believing the lie that it would eventually lead me to become someone worth something. But instead I eventually found myself posing for salacious and tawdry photographers, pretending the required wardrobe of scarcely more than stilettos and a smile wasn't feeding into my shame—or triggering buried memories.

I couldn't pick a healthy friend if life depended on it and had what little I owned stolen from me. Twice. For as bad as I was at choosing friends, I was even worse at choosing boyfriends. On several occasions I found

myself with a Hallmark movie dreamboat (and consequently, the envy of *all* the girls), only to have him turn out to be the kind of man they make Lifetime movies about, cautionary tales of the most disturbing nature.

I chose not to go into any further depth of detail about those experiences because the last thing I want to do is glamourize any of it. I chose to include only this much to stress the fact that while these kind of life experiences might look enviable from the outside, the reality is that on the inside, many who live this way are hollow and broken, longing for something to save them. For Someone to save them. *That* is the accurate description of me in those days.

No matter the high or the low, each relationship, each experience or experiment came at a significant price. And each left me emptier than before. Many of those experiences cost pieces of me that would take years to recover and restore.

But it didn't matter at the time. I never looked at the cost. I didn't see much value in me, so I didn't have much to say when others didn't see it either. A deeply unhappy consequence of all those toxic relationships was that I couldn't even trust the ones who may have been trustworthy. While they didn't deserve it, I lumped them in with those who did or could hurt me.

After my encounters with the boys at school, my friend's father, my uncle and counselor, I pretty much resigned myself to the fact that my greatest value wasn't what was on the inside, but what I had to physically offer and how I looked on the outside. And if I was going to be seen as just a body, then I needed to fool myself into believing I was going to be in control of how that played out.

I was complicit in the exploitation of my own body and my own sexuality, believing the lie that it was empowering, and that instead of being controlled, it put me in control. I had to convince myself that these

were *my* choices in order to live with the consequences of the damage it did to me. But, the most dangerous lies are the ones we tell ourselves. Washed down with enough alcohol and drugs and you can convince yourself of anything. Almost.

DEEPEST REGRETS AND HIDDEN PRIVILEGE

The truth is for all the attention I was getting (for all the wrong reasons), I was terribly lonely and, although I couldn't admit it, I was consumed by shame over the decisions I was making. Yet I felt powerless to stop the cycle. By 18, I looked 25 and felt like I was a thousand years old on the inside... tired of living; tired of others. Tired of myself.

On the outside, there were parts of my life that at times looked glamorous to the untrained eye. Modeling contracts. National performances with highly accomplished artists. Traveling in circles with the rich and famous. But there was nothing glamorous about it. And the longer I stayed in that world the more I compromised myself.

It was all about finding new ways to run. Run from what happened to me. Run from my past. Run from addiction, abortion, failed and abusive relationships. Run from the way I felt. Run from my need for a parent. Run from my shame. And yes, run from God. Eventually, all that running culminated in running from failed attempts at parenting. I don't have words to express the regret I felt (and if I'm being honest, still feel) over how unhealthy I was and how it impacted my kids—particularly my daughter—and how for a time, I handed the legacy of abandonment down to her.

When I found out I was pregnant with my daughter, Ariel, I had delusions about motherhood, I suspect much like those my own mother had. For whatever reason, being naive and 19, I assumed my history, the absence of emotional health and trusted caregivers to emulate it, along

with a lack of being mothered would somehow disappear and become irrelevant when she was born.

I loved her dearly in utero, at birth and beyond. But my love was incomplete and dysfunctional. My priorities were out of whack and I was terrified. Like my own biological mother, I was too broken, too ill-equipped to be a mother. I was still stuck, deeply in need of a mother myself. I had nothing good to offer her and I knew it. The weight of the shame that truth produced was suffocating.

I had the emotional intelligence and relational capacity of an adolescent at best. So, I did what I always did. I ran. And justified my choices as going out to "make a name for myself" and that she was better off without me. On the outside I know I looked like a selfish wild child who shirked her parenting responsibilities in favor of partying and dangerous living. But on the inside, I was terrified and wounded. I don't say that to make excuses for my behavior *nor* to beat myself up. I've come to the place where I can tell the truth about my choices and hold that in tension with the brokenness from which I made those choices. I have learned that both can be and are true.

Still, there is no excuse for hurting your child. Unwittingly, I was setting her up to experience the same kind of abandonment that so deeply wounded me. Like my biological mother before me, and her mother before her, and even back to my great-grandmother, I was incapable of being the mother my daughter needed and deserved.

My lack of ability to parent came at a cost to both of us. She didn't get the healthy mother she needed, and I missed out on many years of my daughter's life.

The shame over that had me spiraling for years and continuing to make terrible decisions to affirm the low worth I saw in myself. When I became pregnant with my son, Alex, five and a half years later, I still wasn't

the mother I needed to be. But the tiniest bit of a maturity and the faintest call toward emotional health wouldn't allow me to make the same mistakes again. When he was born, I had done enough healing that I was able to be better. Still, I had a *long* way to go.

I had begun to recognize the generational patterns of abandonment and knew the cycle had to be broken. I had yet to face all the other baggage in my life.

My early adult life was riddled with the markings of a lost and broken person. However, if you would have told me that was my condition, it was more likely I would have punched you in the throat rather than hear the painfully obvious stated out loud. Taking an inventory was a risk I couldn't afford. I thought I could just keep my head down and plow through this thing called motherhood. Foolishly, I thought I could give my son what I didn't have.

My daughter and my son deserved so much more. I did too. But when I knew better, I gave them better. And by the grace of God and their beautiful hearts, forgiveness was granted. Now, they continue their journeys to being different, better than me. And in many ways, they are nailing it! Now, don't hear what I'm not saying. They aren't perfect. And at times I see remnants of patterns from my life and the generations before us. They are each on their own unique journey, fighting their battles as a result.

The difference is they have me with them to help them recognize it, support them and offer my experiences, and what I know to be true in our family and what it looks like to heal and grow beyond the generations before them. In so many ways, I see them growing beyond where I was at their age. For that, I am grateful. But I do not minimize the struggles they have gone through, nor the struggles they face presently. And I am right here to face it all with them.

I pray that what they now see in me and what God has redeemed in my life gives them hope and encouragement. Perhaps their motivation in life is because they have vowed not to be like I was no matter what. In either case, I feel nothing but joy over the changes they're seeking in their own lives, and the unbelievable privilege of getting to be a part of it. The cycle is breaking.

YOUR TURN: Reflect. Engage. Write.

This is another opportunity to journal about what you just read in this section. What came to mind as you read this section?

Have you struggled with shame, or regret over decisions you've made that impacted your children, or people you love?

What steps have you taken to work through those emotions?

If you have experienced a "turning point" in your story, take a moment to write about it. If not, what steps do you think would help you reach your turning point?

(Maybe reading this book is the beginning of your turning point!)

CHAPTER 14 A Glimpse of God

JESUS FREAKS

In my quest to "plow through motherhood" I tried my hand at getting involved in a few churches. (Which, if I'm being honest, was another attempt to not face what was going on inside of me. I thought I could "cover it up" with Jesus.) Early on, it didn't go well. I went to a couple of churches where I decided to take a risk and let people know a little bit about me. *Very* little. With their judgments and conditional acceptance, they quickly proved that church wasn't a safe place either. Yet there was a nagging piece of me that didn't want to give up on church completely. In hindsight, it was less about not giving up on church and more about not giving up on Jesus.

I think there was always a part of me, even if not in my immediate conscious mind, that somehow knew if I was going to really make it, God would have to be in the picture. Perhaps a part of me remembered Sister Debbie (a special teacher at my grade school) and the bright spot she was in my life. She made me believe that God loved me and would be there for me.

I realize that isn't the case for everyone.

Unbeknownst to me at the time I made one of my many moves, it was God who changed things for me (geographically speaking) and brought me to live in a condo with a church right in its back yard. I'm not kidding! You literally opened the back gate in my yard, walked across a small parking lot, and arrived at the steps of the church!

It was a quirky place, with people from many walks of life. To say they were a little charismatic in their worship would be an understatement. But they *really* loved Jesus. Not in a showy or fake way, albeit in a loud and what I thought at the time, slightly "out there" way. Best of all, they expressed their love for Jesus in the way they loved people. It wasn't long before they showed me that they loved me too.

They flung wide-open the doors of their church and many of them did the same with the doors of their homes. It was like a salve for my soul. It wasn't long before I was, in a manner of speaking, taken in by a couple who were formerly part of a motorcycle gang, Sal and Vic. And when I say, "motorcycle gang," if you're conjuring up scenes in your mind from some of the more colorful portrayals by Hollywood of motorcycle gangs, you're closely accurate to the life this couple lived BC (that's "Before Christ"). Their past aside, they *loved* Jesus. And they loved me.

While they did it in a covert sort of way, I think Sal and Vic sort of parented me. They helped me to be a parent. They planted seeds in my life for which I will always be grateful. But I struggled to completely trust them, unconvinced that I was redeemable. They sensed my hesitation and they never pushed me.

It was in this church with these kind people that I prayed my "first" Prayer of Salvation. For those of you who don't know, that's a prayer asking for God's forgiveness, acknowledging Jesus as Lord and accepting Him as

your personal Savior. But I prefer the sweet way they say it in many kids' church services: *I asked Jesus into my heart and to be my forever friend.*

And I meant it.

But the circumstances of my life, my past hurts and trauma, and the ghost of the wrong Jesus from my childhood haunted me. The dysfunction that went generations deep in my family overwhelmed that moment of surrender. I couldn't trust it. It would take a lot more therapy and many more encounters with this real Jesus before I would find the healing my heart and soul were searching for.

As much as I wanted to stay and rest in these new relationships, I couldn't allow myself to trust them. Even with their love, I still felt hollow inside. I still believed I wasn't enough. My heart wanted to fully embrace this new life and love I was experiencing, but the shame of where I had been and what I had done worked hard to convince me that it wasn't real.

I hadn't told anyone about being molested as a child by a friend's father. I hadn't shared much about the darkness that plagued my past and haunted my present. I think there was a part of me that believed all of that disqualified me from ever being fully loved, so I could never let myself be fully known. I just showed people the parts I thought might be loveable, flawed as they were. Even though my heart yearned for more experiences like my time with Sal, Vic and the rest of the people at that little church, I didn't trust it. Eventually, I left.

I slid back into old habits quickly and rekindled some relationships that offered a counterfeit filler to the void I felt in my life after leaving the church. But the void felt bigger then. Having had the beautiful experience I did at the church, I knew what I was settling for wasn't the *real thing*. I was miserable. And that misery led to a few more bad decisions before the tide began to turn. But first, I had to go through two more abusive relationships and a severing of ties with my biological mother

and brothers before I would intentionally and intensely seek the healing I needed. It was during that time when the sense of self I was attempting to create without dealing with my past burst into a thousand jagged pieces—something that only a Divine intervention would be able to put back together.

In Part Seven, we will visit a bit more in depth my whole perspective on "Jesus and a Therapist," but for now, I just wanted to throw out there that there is no "formula" for your healing or whether you allow God to be involved or not. (But I sure hope you do.) Despite the rough beginnings, church was where I met the first people in my life (with the exception of Sister Debbie, of course) who would serve as living examples of how God could work in my life... *if* I would let Him.

TURNING TIDES ON A SHIFTING SEA

It wasn't until my youngest son was two years old that everything started to take a more permanent shift in my life. Not in an intentional or controlled way. Because, in what universe would I have had the skills to do something in an intentional and controlled way? Instead, imagine the sort of chaos that drives a person to their knees. Literally. Now, add to that chaos, teetering on the verge of being homeless, jobless, car-less and pretty much hopeless. Now, multiply that by a factor of ten and you'll be close to describing the state my life was in. Later (much later), I would recognize all of that as the most beautiful blessing I never asked for.

I was in yet another abusive relationship, cohabitating with a man 20 years my senior and quickly reaching the conclusion that the only interests he was looking out for were his own. I couldn't trust him and his constant attempts at gaslighting (I didn't know what that was at the time, although it *felt* incredibly familiar. In case *you* don't know what *gaslighting* is, here's a great definition from Britannica. *"Gaslighting is an elaborate and insidious technique of deception and psychological manipulation,*

usually practiced by a single deceiver, or "gaslighter," on a single victim over an extended period. Its effect is to gradually undermine the victim's confidence in his own ability to distinguish truth from falsehood, right from wrong, or reality from appearance, thereby rendering him pathologically dependent on the gaslighter in his thinking or feelings." Now you know. And, having read this far in my story, you also know why it felt so familiar to me).

I was never certain what state our relationship was in, but given we lived in his house, I worked to keep him appeased. After a very ugly, alcohol-infused conversation with him (one in which he informed me he wanted to date other people but still sleep with me), I felt we were at the end. I ran up the stairs and threw myself on the bed. I sat up on my knees, my fists held high and as I shook them towards the sky, I cried out to God, *"I can't do this anymore! Either you kill me, or you take over this life because I can't do this anymore."* Then, I cried myself to sleep.

To my great displeasure, I didn't wake to find the clouds had parted, or that the sun was shining and God had fixed everything, just the way *I* wanted Him to.

But if we're being honest, you and I both know that sometimes you don't get to slay the dragon and live happily ever after—at least not until you come to terms with the fact that the dragon is living inside of you.

YOU CAN'T FIX DECADES OVERNIGHT

I guess you could call what happened that night the beginning of an "awakening." This wasn't a cognitive realization of my dysfunction or recognition of my need for help. It was deeper, more visceral and rawer. That night the weight of all I'd been carrying for most of my life came

rushing over me. It was a full-contact experience, invading me mentally, physically, spiritually and emotionally.

But for as much pain as I was in, I still wasn't fully ready to face what my life had become. Despite that, God took my fist-shaking-prayer seriously that night, and unbeknownst to me, He set to work. It wasn't long before I began to realize that the pain required to change couldn't possibly be greater than the pain of staying the way I was. I knew deep down it was time. I just wasn't sure I could do it. And I certainly didn't know *how.*

The night of the prayer, I could sense the battle. Not the one between me and my boyfriend. One far less tangible, but equally visceral. It was deeper than what was transpiring in my physical existence. The weight was oppressive. The heaviness felt familiar. Dark. The darkness ushered in memories of the past.

I was basically in one of, if not *the* worst relationship of my life and was dependent on him for the roof over my head and the car I drove. I couldn't imagine the path to freedom from there. Yet I knew there wasn't a single reason left to trust that man. I had reached a tipping point that night. While nothing in my situation had changed, *I* was different. Just as in all stories of transformation, there is one particular and powerful incident that sets the world spinning in a whole new direction. I would come to realize that, for me, the direction changed with that prayer.

In the moment, however, I was backpedaling like my life depended on it. Once I realized the weight of what I had said to God, I desperately wanted to take it back. But there my words were. Still hanging in the air between us. Thick with pain and shame and sorrow. With all the risk I took in saying such a prayer, I would like to say that I just left it that way. That I stuck with that original prayer and somehow felt cleansed and ready for change. But sadly, I didn't. ***Not yet anyway.***

I confess that at one point, my pulse quickened at the idea that God could, in fact, choose to kill me as opposed to taking over and changing my life. I wasn't convinced He had any mercy left for me and my antics. My flaw was in judging Him by my own fallible, human standards.

When I caught my breath and the dust settled, I tried to go on like nothing had happened that night. I really wanted God to let me forget the whole messy experience. Well, at least the "kill me" part, anyway. I wasn't convinced that I deserved God's intervention. Oh sure, my head knew all the stuff about "ask and you will be forgiven" and that "God loves you and will help you when ask," but I had also been taught to believe that God would "get you" if you stepped out of line.

Heck, I had even seen *really* bad things happen to *really* good people! Since I didn't consider myself to be a good person, I could only imagine what God might see fit to do to me. While my confidence in His love for me was thin, my confidence in my ability to change was even thinner.

But none of my humanness deterred His intervention in my life. He started by orchestrating the bottom falling out of my relationship which, at the time felt like the bottom falling out of my life. Oh, what tender mercies can be disguised as tragedies.

BLESSINGS IN DISGUISE

While I barely eeked out a traditional education, one thing I was intrinsically good at was getting hired at jobs for which I was completely unqualified. I could convince an employer of my abilities despite the lack of their appearance on my sparse (and mostly fictional) resume. Then, once I was in said position, I would work like a fiend to learn *and* excel in my role—especially in roles where I could express my creativity.

I had landed a great job during the chaos of my toxic relationship. It was the one thing I had going for me that was *all mine*.

Because of my creativity (and ability to talk to *anyone)* I was assigned a sales trip to San Antonio. I was stressed about being gone, given the state of things at home, but it was either travel or lose the best job I ever had up to that point. So, I hesitantly boarded the plane with my boss for a three-day trip.

By the end of day one my anxiety was raging. In yet another terrible parenting decision, my boyfriend was supposed to be helping with my son, but he wasn't answering any of my calls. (My daughter was living with her dad's side of the family at the time.) I couldn't concentrate on work and my boss was getting frustrated. By the middle of day two I broke down and called my neighbors, a sweet Christian couple, Sandy and Joel, who occasionally watched my son for me. Sandy answered on the second ring.

"Hey Sandy, it's Gina. I'm trying to get in touch with T and he isn't answering. I'm getting a little worried. Would you mind checking on him and Alex?" I really didn't want to involve her, but I felt I had no choice.

"Alex is here with us, honey. T dropped him off yesterday afternoon," she said in a quiet, compassionate voice. I could tell she wasn't giving me the whole story. *Why hadn't she called me?*

"Oh!" I exclaimed, quickly trying to quell the panic in my voice. Fearing I would lose my job if I asked to be sent home, I tried to downplay the situation and offered to send someone to pick up my son.

"No, no. We're having a great time! He's safe here. Tomorrow will be just fine." There was silence for an extra beat while Sandy worked to take the "chipper" in her voice up a notch. "Do you need us to pick you

up from the airport?" And just like that, I knew that what little home life I had was no more.

In my most grateful voice I responded, "Thanks so much, Sandy. No. I left my car at work so I'll just ride with my boss back to the office and be home as soon as I can." I'm confident she heard the relief and gratitude in my voice as her tone brightened.

"Oh...OK. Well... if you *do* need something, please call. Anything, OK honey? We're happy to help in any way we can." It felt like she was willing me to know something telepathically that she couldn't say out loud. I was already late to my next meeting, so I quickly chatted with Alex (who was in fact having the time of his life) and ended the call.

When I got off the plane and back to the office that next day, any remnants of my life and relationship with T were buried underneath a pile of rubble—solidified by the realization that my car was nowhere to be found.

"My car is *gone*!" I tried to quell the panic rising in me. In a rush, I blurted out "I think my boyfriend took my car. And I don't think I have anywhere to live." I asked my boss for time to collect my son and figure out what I was going to do. It was a Wednesday, and he graciously offered to give me the rest of the week off.

A friend picked me up and together we picked up Alex. The boyfriend had hidden my car and my things and refused to give any of it back until I paid him back the money he had originally "given" me for the car. At least he had the decency to pack a couple large suitcases of mine with some of Alex's clothes and his favorite toys and leave them at Sandy's.

There I was. No car. No belongings. No home. No plan. No idea what I was going to do. And it was the best thing that could've happened to me.

Although I couldn't see it at the time, God had begun a work in my life. He showed up time after time in the most creative and covert ways imaginable. Some of those ways were more obvious in the moment than others.

With the help of friends, and by the grace of God, a temporary plan was hatched, complete with a wonderful daycare for my son. (Like I said, God showed up in all kinds of places.) It was a deeply painful and confusing time in my life. But it was also a time of great relief too. It's hard to explain, but that ending in my life was really a beginning. Funny how we get those mixed up sometimes.

Perhaps in most stories, this would be the place where the protagonist recognizes God's provision and learns of His unfailing love, gets her act together and goes on to honor God with the rest of her life. But in my story? We weren't quite there yet.

It wasn't that I hadn't learned *anything* from the experience. Some things were different. But I still lived in reactionary mode. Everything I did was to make it through the day. And when I couldn't, I would still self-medicate. While I had stopped doing drugs, I still turned to alcohol or the next relationship with someone who seemed to hold the promise of making it all better. What's that they say about the definition of insanity? Continuing to do the same thing and expecting a different outcome? That pretty much summed up my life.

But God was patient with me. Looking back, I can see those failed relationships were more examples of His mercy. As the seeds that were unknowingly planted by helpful people and even from that fist-shaking, desperate prayer took root, I experienced more and more awareness and more unsettledness with the condition of my life. The awareness came in small doses, accompanied by emotionally corrective experiences (more on those in Part Six) that helped to build my sense of faith and trust. They

were the experiences that would eventually provide the grace I needed to face my story in small doses, to heal and grow.

These experiences and relationships also helped me deconstruct and unlearn some things to make room for the healthier life I wanted to create. In the words of Richard Rohr, "Sometimes, we have to leave home to go home."

PART FOUR
Finding Father

CHAPTER 15

Missing Pieces

CATHY'S GIFT

From the time I was reintroduced to my biological mother, most of our conversations centered around subjects she was comfortable with. She liked to talk about our future together, offering very parental advice, and reliving the handful of memories we had accumulated in our brief time back in each other's lives. She also liked to tell me about what I was like as a baby, even though her time with me then had been brief.

Looking back, I can appreciate all of that now, her desire to cling to the good and attempt to establish or validate herself as my mother. And, perhaps, to do her best to offer me something positive.

Sadly, I was too conflicted about all the different dynamics to really see that. I think at a deeper level, I didn't really trust much of what she said. I had no foundation to stand on with her. Most of what she said about me as a baby left me confused. *"If I was such an adorable, perfect baby,"* I thought, *"then why did you decide you didn't want to keep me?"*

In my young mind, that was a legitimate question.

It was rare when Cathy left space for silence or room for me to share how I was feeling. Asking her questions pertaining to my adoption or what her life was like when I was a baby were treated as incendiary.

But occasionally, she would allow me to express what was on my mind. I can imagine how terrifying that must've been, risking that I would ask after something she was unprepared to face.

In the times I visited her, Cathy loved to take car rides together at night. It was her way of getting time alone with me and time away from the stress of her marriage and my brothers. One special, late night ride in her minivan, around the time I was eleven and a half, she left more space than usual for me to say how I felt and what I was thinking, and even to ask questions. On that night, the stars aligned, ever so perfectly, to allow me to ask my biological mother the mother of all questions.

"Hey, Mom?" (It was my decision to call her Mom. "Cathy" didn't feel quite right.) "What can you tell me about my *real* dad?"

"My real dad." My choice of words spoke volumes about my level of maturity. And possibly, said more about how I felt toward Ernie and David. The words communicated "whoever these guys are, they certainly *can't be* my *real* dad." Real dads don't act like that. Right? I was too young and too desperate for acceptance from a father, so I couldn't recognize that the guy who left her (and me) might not be qualified to be called my *real dad* either.

Clearly Cathy was unprepared to discuss it further. She did what she often did to avoid hard things with me. She cried. It was like her super-power. Her way of deflecting and protecting herself. Her voice weakened by tears, she attempted to deflect my prodding. "Honey, that was such a difficult time in my life." She talked about how painful the

subject was for her. And even though I felt the pull to care for her in the moment, I could not be deterred from my mission.

Once Cathy realized I would not abandon my quest for information, she miraculously was able to compose herself and seemed to be considering something. Her brow furrowed and it felt as though she was debating with herself. She waited so long before responding I thought she was going to simply move on without acknowledging my request. Then slowly, Cathy, my Mom, gave the most selfless and motherly response she could provide.

With a sigh that seemed to carry the weight of the world she said, "OK honey, your biological father's name is Dean Payne. But honestly, babe, he may not be your father. I'm not totally sure. I wish I could tell you something different. I'm sorry."

OK, it was *mostly* motherly.

As I contemplated the consequences of her words, Cathy interrupted my thoughts with what I now look at as an attempt at damage control. "You know," she began slowly, "he met you once when you were about six weeks old. He held you, said 'she's not mine' and handed you back to me." Her voice dripped with what was either disdain or pain—most likely, both.

She watched my face quietly. I felt the swell of emotions threaten to overtake me as her words settled in, but instead, I made a conscious effort to swallow them whole. Given that I was conditioned to care for my caregivers, my efforts to emotionally distance myself were partly to prevent Cathy from feeling pain, and partly because I didn't feel safe to express what I was thinking or feeling.

My reply was simple. "Thanks for telling me, Mom." Then I turned the topic to something she was better equipped to handle. *Shopping.*

I'll never know if Cathy told me that painful story to try and prevent me from asking more questions, or if she said it because it was true—perhaps, both. Still, to this day, no matter how hard I try, I can't imagine any outcome in which it would be a good idea to tell a child a story like that, one that most assuredly would hit at their very identity. In either case, I didn't want her to see that it affected me.

After her story that night, I told myself I didn't care who this guy was. The more I thought about it, the more I began to think she made the name up anyway. I mean, seriously. *Dean Payne?* Sounded like a character in a 1950's movie. But deep down inside, the little girl in me longed and hoped for a day when this person, if he was real, would be known to me and want to know me in return.

RISKING WOUNDS

When I began working on this book you now hold in your hands, I sought the advice of a professional editor in the industry who made mention of at least trying to explore my family from my biological father's side. This frustrated me, understandably so, as I had done a tremendous amount of work around the impact of fatherlessness in my life. I didn't really care to create more opportunities for pain that, at the time, seemed unnecessary. But God had a different plan.

As far back as my knowledge of being adopted goes, there has been a part of me that wanted to know who my biological father was. Perhaps the desire to know him was intensified because of the unhealthy relationships I had with the fathers and father-figures in my life (Ernie, Dave, Corky, etc.). At the same time, my experience of being rejected by fathers and father-figures, coupled with the alleged rejection by my biological father when I was a baby, sort of felt like a "three strikes and you're out" kind of thing. So, I worked hard to convince myself that I neither wanted nor needed a father.

But my conversations about the book warred with my seemingly logical reasons to avoid the quest for my elusive, biological father. I felt a new resolve to try to find him, and it wouldn't leave me alone. Sitting here now, having the privileged view from "the other side," I should say that it was *God* who wouldn't leave me alone. God was using my circumstances to call me into a deeper relationship with Him. Admittedly, it was a call I was less than willing to answer at times. In many ways, the idea of trusting God, *another* Father-figure, was an idea that terrified me.

After all, I had plenty of reasons that looked perfectly reasonable on paper to feel I couldn't always trust that God would protect me or that He would work things out in the least painful way.

Then there was the possibility that I *would* find my biological father and he would be a terrible person, someone I was better off not knowing. What if he was dead? Or the worst possible scenario? That he was wonderful!—but would have no interest in having a relationship with me. Each hypothetical situation I conjured up was enough on its own to give me a legitimate reason to take a hard "pass" on the quest.

My history had prevented me from entertaining the possible scenario that he could be wonderful *and* want a relationship with me.

As for the act of inexplicable trust it would take for me to jump into this journey with God? The conversations between us sounded something like this...

Me: "OK, I *think you're asking me to pursue finding this guy. But I've been down this road before. Remember? It ended with a little too much wine and a pint of Ben and Jerry's Cherry Garcia, lots of tears, way too many F-bombs? Oh! And a vulnerability hangover the size of Texas. Been there. Done that. And I don't want to feel that way again. Ever."*

God: *"Yes, I remember. I was there. And I don't want that for you either."*

Me: *"God, this is really scary."*

God: *"I know. Trust me."*

Me: *"Yeah, still not sure... But I'm telling you now, I can't handle another 'Dad-shaped' disappointment."*

God: *"That makes sense. Now let's get started. And Gina, just so* you know? *I will always be your Father."*

All of that might sound a little crazy to some of you. There's a chance you think both of those voices belonged to me. But I know different. And here's why...

Immediately after this conversation, I felt something different—nothing creepy or hyper-spiritual about it, just a feeling in my gut that I attribute to God. Y'all have probably "followed your gut" at one time or another in your life. Well, I believe the driver of *my* "gut" is God and he led me to sign up for a membership with Ancestry.com and within mere moments I was looking at a family tree from my mothers' (Judy's and Cathy's) side of the family. I was holding out hope that a connection could be made with someone who had intel on my biological father. Surely Cathy must have told someone in the family who he really was.

On Ancestry, when there is a connection to follow, you will see a little leaf appear. The leaf is like a clue saying "Follow me! There's more information to learn!" I was surprised to see one so quickly. When I clicked on the name attached to the leaf, it gave me the option to send the person a message. "Why not?" I thought. "Might as well dive into this thing headfirst."

Hi Katie-

My name is Gina Birkemeier. My biological mother was Cathy and my adopted mother was Judy Frank. I think there's a chance you and I might be related as your name popped up when I was searching information on my family. I would love the opportunity to connect and see if we have some people in common.

If you would like to continue the conversation, you can reach me through this site or at my personal email listed below.

All the Best,
Gina

Nothing too deep or emotional. I kept it light and tried hard not to have any expectations. After all, I didn't want to scare the poor woman! To my surprise, a reply came quickly.

Hi Gina! Thanks for the message. Yes, we are related, and I know exactly who you are. You were in my Aunt's wedding when you were little!

And just like that, in 27 little words, I was known. I had family—a connection to my roots.

This was my *cousin* Katie. And, although I had no recollection of being in the wedding she referenced (despite her photographical evidence to prove I was, in fact, there), this would be an important connection in more ways than I could've imagined that day. So far, that "trusting God" thing was working out for me.

That email exchange set off a whirlwind of deepening the connection. Talking to her. Meeting her. Looking into her face and seeing a deep resemblance to my own—and to my kids. She's so lovely. Sage-like,

really. Wise beyond her younger-than-me years. She led me to other family members who were excited to learn that Katie and I had connected and who were willing to answer questions about my mother(s) and about me.

Even more generous were the photos she and other family members shared. The photos were proof of the childhood I had been so unsure of, like filling in the pieces missing from a puzzle. It was difficult to hear many of the answers and admittedly, it put me back in therapy for a little while. But some of those stories connected dots for me.

While these new-found connections presented some new challenges and even some new hurts, they also created a space of healing for my soul—in part, because of their immediate love and acceptance towards me. However, while I will always be grateful for that experience, none of it got me any closer to finding my biological father. In fact, none of them knew anything about him. It was a loving gesture that they wanted to help me and were sincerely disappointed that they couldn't. But since this whole "trusting God" thing seemed to be working out, I decided to keep going on the journey.

I asked God for more clarity and direction on finding my biological father. I was working hard not to *tell* the Great Divine how I felt this whole thing should play out, but I couldn't resist throwing in my two cents on what I felt He should *not* let happen.

But since I hadn't received the information I most hoped for from my "new" relatives, and consequently had come up against a lot of dead ends in the quest, I reluctantly asked God if He was closing the door on this whole adventure.

"OK God, am I supposed to keep pushing on what feel like closed doors here? If so, I'm gonna need you to help. And if I'm not? I'm gonna need

even *more* help to understand why you led me on this whole journey to begin with." *Amen.*

As much as I wanted answers, I didn't *really* want them if they were only going to cause pain without purpose. Pain with purpose? That I could be OK with. But not pain that served no greater good.

For all of my self-deception about how much I was allowing God to be in control, that space in the journey revealed just how little of my vise-like grip on the situation I had actually released. He was about to show me how much better the ride would be if I let Him take the wheel.

CHERYL: A *RE*-INTRODUCTION

I felt another shift when I prayed that prayer for help. My inner control freak was slightly in check. Some of my fears subsided. Or perhaps morphed in their shape and size. Nonetheless, they weren't the oppressive weight they had been before. While I still felt uncertain, mostly I felt free. It's funny what you can make room to discover within the regions of your own memories when you feel free.

Searching the scattered archives of my memory, replaying the information I had, a name popped into my mind. *Cheryl.* (Actually, it was her *whole* name, but I'm going to leave that out of print.) It came so fast and so clear, I had to stop and double check myself, making sure the name was real. Then I remembered that it was definitely real. Cheryl was Cathy's best friend.

As a bonus, I also remembered Cathy telling me she had known Cheryl since *high school.*

I began my search where I was sure to find a fountain of accurate information. *Facebook.* Quicker than you can say "stalker," her image

popped up right in front of my eyeballs. And I *remembered* her! I took a deep breath and looked up to the sky. "OK, that was definitely You, God." I sent a brief, private message to Cheryl and then, I waited.

I think I refreshed and checked my Instant Messenger at least 978,643 times those first couple of days. Finally, the little icon at the bottom of the message I sent her had changed color, indicating she had read it. Or, she had at least seen it. Still, no reply.

I played a thousand scenarios in my mind. I wondered if Cheryl had even stayed in touch with Cathy. Did she know that I was not in communication with my mother and brothers? That my relationship with her never found its footing after so many starts and stops. I wondered if Cathy had told her about my decision to separate from the toxicity of my brothers and stepfather. I wondered if Cheryl knew about my brothers' battles with drugs and alcohol (an inheritance from our mother's side) or how violent they had become (an inheritance from their father), evidenced by assault charges, time in jail and many casualties in their wake. Was she aware of the sheer insanity? The alleged ties to drug cartels and other malevolence. Was it possible that Cathy had told her that she viewed my separation from my brothers and her husband as a separation from her? Had Cheryl taken Cathy's side?

Had she known that Cathy died several years before from complications due to diabetes? Or that she was preceded by one of my brothers who died the year before in a fatal (and suspicious) car crash? All the darkness swirled in my mind. I prayed I would not be the bearer of such terrible news to this woman who, at least at some point, had been Cathy's dearest friend.

My brain tried to make up a thousand stories for why she hadn't replied. I worked hard to thwart rejection and shame in their attempts to overtake me. I fought back the idea that trusting God with this whole "father thing" was a mistake.

But sometimes, grace wins and you catch your breath just long enough to see a light shining amidst the storm. I had yet another frantic conversation with God, but at the end of it, I felt like I could trust him. I believed it. I believed *Him.*

That day, I stopped refreshing and checking my IM every 90 seconds, and (somewhat begrudgingly) yielded to God's control. And what do you know? The next day, I received a brief reply, saying she would welcome the opportunity to meet.

I steadied myself and typed my reply.

> *"Thanks, Cheryl. I would really like that too. Maybe we could meet for coffee or possibly lunch? I want to be honest though, I have some questions I would like to ask you. Given that my mom is no longer with us, I'm hoping you will consider answering my questions with any information you may have felt the need to keep secret while she was alive."*

I decided to assume she already knew about my mother's death and hope that the news didn't come as a shock. It was a bold ask, I know. But for some reason I didn't feel sheepish about my request.

On the day of our meeting, I prayed all the way to the restaurant. I had also prayed in the shower, while putting on my makeup, at the store the night before, during a conversation with the clerk at the gas station on the way there, in the parking lot as I walked across it... you get the picture. I literally prayed all the way through the doors of our meeting spot!

As I walked through the heavy glassed, double doors of the restaurant, Cheryl stood. She rushed to hug me, tears in her eyes. It had been decades since she last saw me, but she didn't even wait for clarification that I was me. She knew. I'm guessing because I have my mother's eyes.

She held me for a long moment, then pushed me back at arm's length, holding my shoulders as she examined my face. The familiarity of my resemblance to my mother evident in her expression. Seeing the tenderness in her eyes, it was hard for me to keep the emotion out of my own expression, and before I could stop them, the tears flowed.

"I am so glad you found me." She whispered.

Before our backsides hit the bench-seats, Cheryl began peppering me with all sorts of questions. I had plenty of my own questions too. She wanted to know all about me, and I wanted to know all about my biological mother. At the suggestion of Cheryl, we decided to leave the restaurant and head to her home, only five minutes from the restaurant. There, for the next *six hours*, time stood still as she shared memories and photos of my mom and told me things I never knew. Some of the things she told me were completely different versions of stories that were told to me by family. Cheryl took every opportunity she could to remind me that my mother loved me. That wasn't something I was totally ready to believe. But I believe that Cheryl believed it. And I think my mom believed it too. So, I decided in that moment, that could be enough for me.

The afternoon flew by, overflowing with laughter and tears. I left with a greater sense of who my mother was and an appreciation for some of her more audacious qualities, exhibited in stories like the one I'm calling "A Hard Day's Night."

A HARD DAY'S NIGHT

Cathy had an intense relationship with music. She couldn't carry a tune if she had a bucket to put it in, but she knew how to write moving lyrics and she knew how to "tell" someone how they should sound. For her, it was like life had a soundtrack, every event memorialized by its connection to some song or lyric.

She used music to escape, express herself, and even motivate her. When she couldn't find a song to fit how she was feeling or what she was experiencing, she'd just write a new one. In fact, she wrote a lot of songs and poems throughout her life. She had an affinity for all genres of music and artists, but like most 16-year-olds in 1964, the Beatles were a huge part of the soundtrack of her adolescence. John, Paul, Ringo, and George were constant companions on her journey.

As you read earlier, there was tremendous chaos in Cathy's childhood home. And after her mom, Marie, had died, there was no shortage of turmoil either. Cathy experienced a lot of back and forth from her grandparents' house to her dad's house. Sometimes, that choice was hers and other times it was forced upon her. She was restless, feeling like she didn't quite belong in either place. (Much like I felt bouncing back and forth between Judy and Ernie, and eventually, even to Cathy's.)

During a particularly volatile explosion with her grandparents, she hatched a plan to run away, hoping to leave her own family behind and become a card-carrying member of another, more famous family—George Harrison's family, as in George Harrison of the Beatles.

George's sister, Louise Harrison Caldwell, lived a reasonable distance away in Benton, Illinois, so Cathy decided to show up on her doorstep, tell her tale of woe and beseech them to take her in to the Harrison family. In fact, she had been writing letters to Louise for several months and even getting responses! Apparently, those responses were enough to make her believe that the plan to run away and join the Harrison family was a solid one.

As the story goes, Cathy confidently set out for the bus station in downtown St. Louis, where upon arrival she purchased a ticket and boarded the bus headed for Benton, Illinois, and traveled the 100 miles to where she hoped her future was waiting. I imagine her in Benton, walking right up to Mrs. Harrison-Caldwell's door. "Mr. Caldwell?" She says with tears

in her voice, "I'm Cathy Craig. I've been corresponding with your wife for the past several months. Is she here? And, if it's all right with you, I'd like to know if you would consider letting me stay." She left out the part about wanting to stay forever.

I'm not sure if the Caldwell's were taken aback by the audacity of this bold request from a 16-year-old girl, or perhaps moved to compassion by the chaos that was clearly Cathy's life back in St. Louis. Whatever the motivation, Louise and her husband took my mom into their home. They listened patiently, gave her something to drink, fed her lunch and gently informed her it would be wrong for her to stay with them permanently. They convinced her to give them the name of someone they could contact who would come and get her. Of course, they also promised to keep in touch.

Reluctantly, Cathy gave them my great-grandfather's name and number. Louise called and explained the situation and patiently waited while Tony let the information sink in and ask for directions in broken English.

I have to hand it to her; Cathy wasn't afraid to dream big dreams and then go after those dreams. There was an audacity to her that I've been told I inherited in spades, as did my kids. And speaking of things passed down, I see that trait in my grandkids, too.

There were so many stories shared by Cheryl that day.

Beyond the tales that emphasized my mother's heartbreaks and longings, Cheryl shared captivating and interesting stories of my mother's creativity and charm along with her quick wit and take-no-crap attitude. Each piece of information filled some tiny crack in the story of what made mother uniquely her, and in part, made me uniquely me.

One of the most significant moments came at lunch when I asked her about my biological father.

"Did you ever meet him?" I cautiously asked Cheryl, hoping she would not only remember, but would be willing to part with the information.

"No…" Cheryl replied, her tone apologetic. "Honestly, I'm not sure if I remember his name. Carl maybe? Does that sound right?"

I didn't say anything for a beat, wondering if, given enough space, she would fill it with more information. Sensing I was waiting for her to say more, she continued.

"There was a time where your Mom and I didn't talk. I was settling down, getting married and had just found out I was pregnant. Cathy was still living a pretty crazy life, hanging out with different friends—people I didn't really associate with. We just sort of drifted apart. I saw her a little bit here and there. But we weren't close while she was pregnant with you nor the first few months of your life."

I felt defeat creeping in. But then, I heard it. That still small voice.

"Trust Me."

Unwilling to give up easily, I forced myself to speak before I could convince myself that I shouldn't. I took a deep breath and blurted out the name. The name that sounded made up. The name that my mother had given me all those years ago. The name that haunted me over the years.

"Do you by chance remember her mentioning a guy named Dean? Dean Payne?" I continued quickly before she had a chance to shoot me down. "I'm just wondering, because I seem to remember Cathy telling me that was his name. My *father's* name, I mean."

Cheryl's eyes grew wide. She raised her forearm parallel to the table and held it inches from my face. She pointed to the goose bumps on her arms that forced the tiny hairs to stand at attention as she rapidly

repeated, "That's it! That's him! Oh my gosh, Gina! I have chills!" Her voice shook and I could see tears threatening to spill from the corners of her eyes.

My face grew hot and my eyes began to sting from the tears threatening to spill everywhere despite my resistance. My ears tingled and my heart raced. I adjusted in my seat more for the sake of grounding myself (a technique used for staying present and not being overtaken by my emotions) on the cool faux leather of the booth. It took me a minute to realize I wasn't saying any of the things I was thinking out loud.

"Thank you so much." I said, working hard to keep my voice steady. "Knowing his name will help me tremendously."

I was grateful for the confirmation Cheryl gave. But a little part of me couldn't help but wonder if her deeply emotional reaction was a response to Dean's name jarring a once lost memory, or because she knew it would now be OK to admit she knew his name because Cathy had in fact given it to me herself.

But the thought drowning out all the others was this: *"We may actually have a shot at finding this guy!"*

Just as quickly as I felt hope rising, I could feel something competing. A sense of slipping back into self-protection mode. I wanted to protect myself from feeling any more hurt or betrayal by another "father." Then, right on cue, I felt it again… My heavenly Father, inviting me to trust Him once more.

MEET MY HUSBAND

I was exhausted from crying and laughing and trying to put all the pieces together, but I couldn't wait to share what I had discovered with my

husband. It would take me the better part of the next few days to relay to him all that I had learned from Cheryl. He laughed with me. He cried with me. Eventually, he asked, "OK babe, *now* do you want me to find him?"

I will explain the *"now,"* but first, a little about my husband, Tom.

When I met my husband 21 years ago, I had not done enough work in my story to offer him a fully healed version of myself. I had processed through some portions of my story, coming to terms with my alcohol and drug abuse, and even some of my abusive relationships. I had worked through the parts of my adoption story (that I knew about) up to a certain point. Still, many of the events that had caused me deep pain and shame remained locked away.

So, in lieu of being able to offer him the *healthiest* version of myself, I reinvented myself instead, offering him a bright and shiny version of me. Six months from the day we met we were engaged and eight months from that day, we were married. Having already disconnected from my family by this time, my side of the wedding venue was filled with friends instead. But none of that mattered to me. I had put the past behind me. Or, more accurately, walled it off from my present. I really believed that I had done enough work that I could just move on and build a life with Tom. I didn't want the things of my past infecting my present or my future.

But avoidance is not a strategy for healing. Ironically, I was re-wounding the parts of me that were already wounded and fragile—parts that needed attention, not banishment. The deeper I fell in love with him and his three boys, the more terrified I became to let him know all the details of my past, or admit that there were pieces of my story that even I was unable to recall. But eventually, you have to remove the mask, or you will suffocate beneath it.

Avoidance is not a strategy for healing.

When I finally began to share things with him, he was understandably confused, feeling a bit like a bait and switch had occurred. We fought hard to stay together; his past wounds colliding with mine. More therapy, and more Jesus kept us together and healed us together.

Between us we have five children, and we claim them all as our own. In direct contrast to the stepparent in my story, we have abandoned any terms and postures of the heart which feel like separating his from mine. When Ariel met her brothers, she had a loving stepdad who welcomed her with open arms, always telling her he loves her and always showing it with his actions—another cycle so beautifully broken.

By the time I married Tom, I'd like to say that I had magically become a parenting role-model. Sadly, that wasn't the case. In some ways (OK, in *many* ways), I was flying by the seat of my pants. I tried so desperately to be the polar opposite of my neglectful and uninvolved parents that I became too controlling and I fear, at times, suffocating. I was terrified that some of the things that happened to me would happen to them, so I went way overboard in the amount of parenting I offered. Most of my attempts came as a list of "don't's" in the hopes that I could keep them safe. A lot of the time I was in my head, making sure I was doing the opposite of my parents. Since they under-parented, in many instances, I think I wound up over-parenting.

I worry sometimes that they felt more discipline than love from me (although they say that isn't the case). In my exasperation and woeful inadequacies, my fuse grew short quickly and I was exhausted often. Not to mention the uphill battle of having completely different rules than when they went to visit "their other parents." It took me a while to find the balance. It took time for us to find the balance.

Tom and I have been through more in our 21 years than many couples (and families) experience in 50. It took a lot of humility and a lot of help for us to get to where we are now. We had to let go of so many things we

believed that were harming the both of us. We had to surrender our armor of self-protection and be willing to take the risks to trust. We have learned so much about ourselves and each other. Tom has been and continues to be my greatest corrective experience, and according to him, I have been his as well.

LETTING TOM HELP

Over 20 years ago, Tom had asked me if I wanted him to find my biological father. I politely (and firmly) told him "no." He didn't know my whole story yet, and I had yet to share with him that I had dabbled in detective work a few times myself over the years. I didn't want to relive the shame and rejection and dead ends I encountered with every call I had made—all those failed attempts, not wanting to admit he was *the* guy because it might jeopardize whatever life he had built for himself. Each rejection was a confirmation that fatherlessness would remain my story.

And one day, he asked me again.

The idea of opening myself up to all of that again was daunting. And while the fear was real, what I had experienced that day with Cheryl, and this "*trust Me*" thing I had going with God, made me believe something would be different this time.

"Yes," I said resolutely, "I'm ready."

I could tell he was excited, but he remained calm. "OK. I'm on it," he said with a wink and a smile.

And when my husband says, "he's on it," and wants to make something happen—*well*.

It happens.

Tom didn't say much about his search and, not wanting to risk rejection, I didn't ask. We were business as usual on the home front until one day, a week into his research, he came home, laptop in hand and said, "Hey babe, I think I found him."

For a beat, we just stood there staring at each other. Sensing I was experiencing a little bit of paralysis, he spoke first. "Would you like to see where he lives?" His question snapped me out of my stupor. "Absolutely," I said, holding my breath as he slowly and almost reverently opened his laptop, like it contained the precious secrets of the universe. In some ways, I suppose it did.

CLOSE TO HOME

Tom sat next to me on the couch. Balancing his laptop on his palm, he snuggled in close. Then placed the computer on his lap and pulled up Google maps, "I've investigated several people with the name your biological mother gave you and I can only find one match whose timeline, age and geographical history make sense. This man is also the only person in the state of Missouri, *from* Missouri, with the name *Dean Payne*. From what I can tell, here is his current residence."

Tom put the computer in my lap. The picture in front of me looked like cartoon hills, but as he zoomed in the digital illustration turned into real-life images of trees and water and rooftops. I still wasn't sure what I was supposed to be seeing. He saw the confusion on my face and explained.

"See this right here? This is our new home at the Lake. And this..." He pointed to the water mass, "is the stretch of the Lake in front of our home."

"OK..." I said, hesitantly, not knowing where this was going.

"And this?" He pointed to the top of the hill across the water from our home, enlarging the screen to reveal a rooftop tucked in the thick field of trees atop the hill. "This is where the man who I believe is your father lives."

In case you missed it...

Across the water *from our NEW Lake home.*

The one we had purchased mere months before all this happened. The Lake house that was on the unique island where we'd nearly purchased two other homes over the years, but for one reason or another, those deals fell through. *This* home, however, had become ours through Divine intervention, against inexplicable odds. (When your own realtor says "I can't understand why they accepted your offer... But it's yours!" AND calls it "A God-thing," you can hardly argue.)

Even as I type this, I can feel the tears stinging at my eyes. But the night it happened? It was tears and fears; hope mixing with doubt. I needed Tom to repeat what he said. I wanted so badly to maintain neutrality. *"It's just information, Gina. Stay calm."* I said this to myself over and over; working tirelessly to prevent too much hope from building. History was screaming its cautionary tales in my mind.

But hope remained undeterred.

And the little girl inside me was wide awake. She liked hope better than practicality and she refused to be quiet. (It's taken some time, but I've really grown to love her.) Before I could control it, my heart began to plead with God. "Please let this be him. This must be him! God, everything You've orchestrated, with our Lake home, in this place. How could it *not* be him?!"

I looked over at my husband who was patiently studying my face. I have no idea how long I left him hanging while my mind went wild. But, when I took notice of him again, tears threatened to spill from his eyes too. Once we pulled ourselves together, the obvious question presented itself. *"What now?"*

REINFORCEMENTS

Tom set about the business of compiling a list of potential points of contact for Dean Payne, while I called two members of my family (friends who are like family) to fill them in. These beautiful, warrior women have been constant companions on my journey. These are my "fight in the trenches with you, praying their butt off for you, help you hide the body, ride-or-die friends."

They both said what my heart had feared to say. "This *has* to be the guy! How could it *not* be the guy? It would be just like God to work it out this way." And with everything in me, I wanted to believe them.

Just after my call, Tom shared his list. There weren't many names on it, and none seemed to give clues as to how they were connected to him, save for sharing a last name.

Not knowing who-was-who, I was hesitant to reach out to anyone on the list. I didn't want to freak anyone out or spook anyone away. And if I did and they tipped Dean off, how would he take it? Was he in poor health? Because if he were, a statement like "Hey, I think I'm the daughter you abandoned over four decades ago" could throw a frail person into a serious medical situation!

So, instead of trying to reach out, I did what any normal person would do. I stalked them on Facebook—well, the ones I could find anyway. But in the end, I didn't find much helpful information.

I began to wonder if this, like so many other attempts over the years, would be a dead end leading to another heartbreak.

Feeling more than a little defeated and extremely confused by what God might be up to, I turned on the TV to distract myself, but not before voicing my frustrations to God.

In response, He was suspiciously quiet. I was just plain suspicious.

Moving on with my plan for distraction, I flipped through channels and stumbled upon a show I had never seen before called "Lost Family." Can you guess what it was about? Yep. That's right. The story I stumbled across was about an *adult child* looking for their *biological parent!*

I turned my eyes skyward, convinced this meant something. I realize that might seem strange to you. But listen, if God can use a burning shrub to get Moses' attention when he was a man on the lam, He can certainly use an appropriately timed (and named) TV show to get the attention of a stubborn woman.

Almost immediately, a thought hit me out of nowhere: *"Ask your new friend Karen at the Lake if she knows Dean Payne. She grew up there."*

This I could do. I quickly sent her a text. "Hey friend!" I banged out on my phone, "Do you by chance happen to know a guy by the name of Dean Payne?" I waited. Impatiently.

"Nope. Should I?" came the reply.

Yes, Karen. Yes, you should.

"I know an Erika Payne. Does that help?"

E. R. I. ***K.*** A. That spelling was on the list of possible relatives that Tom had shared with me earlier.

"Maybe?"

"Do you by chance know her parents' names?"

"No. But I can find out." she replied.

While waiting for Karen's new intel to arrive, I got my laptop out and scoured over the lists of names we had compiled in relation to Dean Payne. Many of the same names popped up...*including* Erika. But this time, a new, and seemingly unrelated, name appeared.

Josie Mantle.

"Josie Mantle?" I said out loud, confused by the disconnect in last names. I didn't think much of it, chalking it up to an error in the search. It didn't even dawn on me that this new name could be my answer.

A BREAK IN THE CASE

The next day I heard back from Karen.

"Not sure if I mentioned this yesterday, but Erika is a twin," she said. "Their father's name was Dick. He passed away a while back. Their mom's name is Josie. She's a real estate agent here at the Lake and, from what I hear, very well-liked and respected. Unfortunately, her last name isn't Payne. No one remembers what it is. Erika and her sister are really sweet girls, though. I'll keep digging. I'm sure someone around here knows their mom's last name."

JOSIE?! I couldn't believe it.

"Is her last name *Mantle?*" I asked, apprehensively.

"Oh, I think that's it," she shouted. "Wait… How did *you* know that?"

I finally gave in and told Karen the reason behind my original request.

"Well…that guy I asked you about? Dean Payne? There's a chance that he might be my father."

There was a beat of silence. Then Karen spoke rapid fire, *"Oh my GOSH! How EXCITING!"* While I appreciated her enthusiasm, I wasn't quite ready to join her in the celebration. So, I thanked her for her help, and asked her to please keep our conversations confidential. She was happy to oblige and asked if I would mind keeping her posted. I happily agreed. Now that the cat was out of the bag, it was kind of nice to have someone else closer to the situation to share things.

Because of her job, it was easy enough to find Josie's contact information. But before I went any further out on that limb, I placed a call to *our* real estate agent, Paula, at the Lake to confirm Josie was as nice as she was rumored to be. Fortunately, the rumors were true, and while she admitted she didn't know her well, Paula said Josie was a "wonderful person."

That was all I needed. I tapped the number in as quickly as possible. I prayed that the call would be a success, that this woman would *not* think I was a loon or hang up on me, and that God would ultimately make a way for this to be *the* lead to my biological father.

As my internal conversation with God continued, I was completely tuned out to the ringing of her phone. So, I was caught a little off guard when she answered.

"This is Josie." Bright and pleasant. Just as I had hoped.

"Hello Josie? My name is Gina Birkemeier. We don't actually know each other, but the reason I'm calling is because I think there's a chance you and I may be related to the same person."

"Oh!" Her tone understandably surprised and hesitant. "OK...and *who* is that we are talking about?" She seemed more curious than anything. Still bright and pleasant. Certainly, open to what I was saying.

"Well, are you by chance related to a Dean Payne?"

Josie couldn't see it, but I was squeezing my eyes closed tightly and scrunching my nose as I held my breath, waiting for her response.

"Yes. As a matter of fact, I am! He's my brother-in-law." Her tone relaxed even more as she realized I wasn't trying to scam her in some way. "May I ask how you think you may be related to him?" This time, her voice was rich with curiosity.

"Sure.... *(breathe Gina, breathe)* I think he might be my... my father." There it was. All my cards on the table.

"Oh! Wow! OK. And, um, what did you say your name was again?!"

There was the shock I was expecting. Before I could say much more than repeating my name, Josie quickly added that, unfortunately, she was walking into a meeting and had to get off the phone. "But!" she added quickly, "you can call me back. How about in an hour?"

"How about I give you an hour and a half?" I wanted to make sure she had plenty of time to finish whatever she had on her schedule.

"Sounds great! I'll talk to you then." And after the longest hour and a half of my life, I called her back. It was such a relief when Josie answered on the first ring.

I spent the next 45 minutes answering her questions. "Why do you believe Dean could be your father?" And "How old are you...if you don't mind my asking." It was evident she was attempting to put the pieces together to assess how this might impact Dean and his family.

Josie gave me the opportunity to ask several questions of my own as well. Almost immediately we began to exchange pictures via text.

Fortunately for me, while not related by blood, Josie and I share the 'driven gene' and she wasted no time in offering to meet with Dean herself to discuss our conversation and "feel the situation out." She was willing to let him know about me and to share the pictures I had sent of myself, my family and my biological mother. I gratefully said yes, hoping she would be able to open doors of communication that might be difficult to open as a stranger.

It wasn't long after we hung up that Josie sent me more pictures of Dean and the rest of their family. Later I would discover she had contacted her daughters and asked them for photos, but refused to tell them why she wanted them. I was certain I could see a strong resemblance between them and myself. I even showed them to my husband and a couple friends who said they could see it too.

Just as I began to wonder how long it would take for Josie to arrange a meeting with Dean and what his reaction would be, the phone rang.

"Hi Gina! It's Josie. I'm meeting with Dean today at 2:30. I will call you afterwards. But if he wants to talk to you, can I give him your number?" It was already 10 a.m.! I couldn't believe it was all happening so fast.

"I, I guess so. Sure. Yes. Please feel free to give him my number." Stumbling in my reply because, oddly enough, I hadn't thought that far into the plan.

I did a lot of clock-watching that day along with a lot of texting and calling out to the cavalry (my hubby and my closest friends) to join me in a bit of nail biting and prayer. The one bright spot of distraction in the day was that my friend Shelly was taking me to my doctor's appointment that afternoon to check on how my broken foot was healing. The appointment just so happened to be at 2:30. I barely remember what happened in the appointment. I could feel myself on the verge of tears most of the day.

After my doctor's appointment, Shelly took me out for an early dinner and a bit more distraction. While eating was a challenge, having her there to process and help hold the weight of all I was feeling was a gift. Still, I had a hard time keeping my eyes off the clock. Especially since it was three and a half hours past the time that Josie and Dean were scheduled to meet.

Every scenario under the sun was going through my mind and only one or two that were positive. After nearly *four hours*, Josie finally called around six and launched into the news she had to share.

"Well! I just finished meeting with Dean. And he remembers your Mom. Spoke so fondly of her. He was quiet for a while but admitted that he wondered if the daughter Cathy had was his. Dean didn't go into too much detail about that. But he looked at your pictures and said he saw a family resemblance too, just like I did. You really look like a McAllister." Dean's mother's maiden name.

She paused and waited for my response. Tears were silently streaming down my face and even though I wanted to say something, I couldn't find the words or catch my breath enough to speak them if I could.

I finally eked out some words.

"Excuse me please, while I pull myself together."

She waited patiently for me to collect myself before she continued with her report.

"Dean said he was going to go home and talk to his wife. He said once he had a chance to do that, he would call you. I'm not sure when that will be as she's been ill recently. But if you don't hear from him in the next few days, please call me back, OK?" Her kindness overwhelmed me.

"OK, I will. Thank you so much for all you've done, Josie. I'm grateful you answered the phone the second time and so grateful for your willingness to step into this." I had abandoned my attempts at keeping tears at bay.

We hung up and I sat in the passenger seat of Shelly's car, letting the tears flow. Words failed me. Internally, I argued with hope. My mind was flooded. I was overwhelmed.

The remainder of the evening, I wrestled between opening myself up to the possibility this could work out and the possibility that I was facing a three-strikes-and-you're-out in the father department.

I would love to tell you I immediately took the whole thing to God, resting in the perfect peace that He would work it all out for my good. But I can't. Oh sure, I talked to God *about* it. Even said things like "I trust You Lord." And while that was mostly true, I'll admit to you (and to myself) that I also didn't. The tough girl in me fought hard to go into self-protection mode. And at times, she won. But something deeper kept fighting for space. Something that kept telling me it was going to be all right.

Somewhere between crying, numbing out with TV, praying, talking to Tom and wrestling with my emotions, my chaos was interrupted by my cell phone ringing. I looked at the screen and saw the area code for the Lake. I knew it was Dean.

I swiped to accept the call and as calmly and cautiously as I could, pushed out a feeble "Hello?"

"Is this *Gee-na*?" a sweet voice on the other end of the line said, drawing my name out like he didn't want to let it go from his lips.

"Hi. Yes, it is. Is this Dean?"

"Yes," he said softly with a sheepish sort of laugh, "I don't really have anything planned for what I want to say but I just wanted to call you. I didn't want to wait or keep you waiting." He spoke with gentle emotion in his voice, but emotion toward what? It was too soon to tell.

For the next 45 minutes, we talked. About him and his family. About me and mine. We talked about my biological mother. We talked about the Lake and about Josie. He mentioned the family resemblance he saw. And of course, we talked about the seemingly impossible "coincidence" that we'd just purchased a home *right across the water* from him. We chatted about the weather and a variety of inconsequential things too.

The conversation had some lulls but mostly we both kept working to fill any silence that dared to seep in. Perhaps we just wanted to hear each other speak a bit more. Maybe we were looking for clues that would reveal commonalities, markers that indicated we were related.

After chatting for a while, I finally asked the big question I'd been wanting to ask.

"Dean, I would really like to get a DNA test done. I think it would be best to not have any questions in either of our minds. The best way to do that would be for us to be together, in the same location. Would you be open to that?" I had no contingency for if he said "no."

"Sure! I can do that. I can be in St. Louis Thursday." That was eagerness in his voice, I was sure. I felt hope rising to a new level in me. His kindness and easy demeanor with me in the midst of our uncertain situation drew me in,—made me want to know him more.

"You mean the day after tomorrow?" I couldn't keep the shock from my voice.

Dean laughed a little. "Yes, does that work for you?" I'm relatively sure he already knew the answer.

"Um...yes, I think so. I'll just need to call the lab and make sure it works for them. Would you like to meet beforehand and talk a bit?"

"Yes, that would really be good."

"OK, I'll call you tomorrow and let you know what the lab says."

"OK." He seemed to be delaying our goodbye. "It was really nice to talk with you." I thought I heard tears in his voice.

"It was a pleasure to talk to you as well. Thank you for calling." *Ugh, there's that "look how much I have my crap together" voice again. Liar.*

The truth is that the little girl inside me wanted to say "I really hope you're my daddy. Do you hope you're my daddy too?" But in that moment, she needed to stay hidden, protected from any harm that might befall her.

I had to keep her at bay for the moment. She wanted to say things that a daughter would say and hear things that a father would say back. That was far too risky and far too unrealistic for this first call. And I simply couldn't take such a risk.

After getting confirmation from the lab the next day that they could "squeeze us in," I called Dean to let him know we were a go. He said he thought that was great and asked for the address of where I wanted to meet. He said he would call the next day when he got closer to ask for more specific directions. It didn't take long to realize he was an old-school-flip-phone man and in his opinion, GPS was a needless accessory.

Sleep evaded me that night. When I did drift off, my dreams were bizarre. I woke several times with my heart beating out of my chest. My mind wouldn't rest, wondering if Dean would really show. I tried breathing exercises, prayer, visualization, the works. Those were helpful things, but none of them wholly did the trick. The little girl in me who dared to hold on to the dream of a father refused to be lulled to sleep. She was on high alert and damned be anyone who tried to get in her way of fantasizing and fretting about the meeting the next day.

MEETING DEAN

Even though I wasn't supposed to drive because I had a broken foot, I did it anyway and it forced me to put my full attention into something other than meeting Dean.

Not wanting to totally go it alone, I called my girlfriend Julie and asked her to come sit with me at the restaurant. I wasn't sure I trusted myself to keep it together if left alone with only 48 years of questions and longing to keep me company. Julie arrived nearly the same time as me and we quickly found a spot in the back of the restaurant and talked through what was about to go down. The weight of all I carried, made lighter by having her there to help hold it all.

Dean was mostly on time and called me when he pulled into the lot. I told him where to find us in the restaurant which was *way* more crowded

than anticipated for that time of day. When he walked in the door, we instantly locked eyes. He beelined for our table and went straight for a hug and planted a gentle kiss on my cheek.

"That's for you and for Cathy." He said with tears welling in his eyes. I felt tears well up in mine too.

The time Dean and I spent together that day was initially awkward, but good. After nearly an hour, we left and headed for the lab. Once inside, I was far more of a wreck than anticipated. Dean seemed calm, cool and collected. It also helped that the lab tech was wonderful. Aside from her initial confusion about who was who and asking, "where is the child?" when we said we needed a DNA test. *(Awkward.)*

She escorted us to a testing room where we sat on a small bench together. I don't remember much about the process except that Dean picked up on how nervous I was and gently reached over and patted my back—already playing the part of "father."

Not knowing what the outcome of the test would be and having my biological mom's voice ringing in my ears *("I'm not even sure that he's the guy")* made it a challenge to stay present.

When we finished, we asked how long it would take to get results. "Five business days or less. They've already picked up for today, so it won't go out until tomorrow."

Dean and I gave a collective and disappointed "Oh," which our lovely technician picked up on.

"Tell you what," she said cheerfully, "I'm finished for today so how about if I drive this directly to FedEx myself, right now?"

We expressed our gratitude and made a quick exit to let her get on with it.

We had driven over to the lab together, and as we reluctantly discussed getting me back to my car, it became clear that neither one of us was ready for the meeting to end.

"Would you like to go grab a drink and talk a bit more?" I really hoped he would say yes.

"I would really like that." He seemed relieved that I was asking.

We drove the short distance so I could fetch my car and headed just across the street to a café. I had to giggle a bit watching him puzzle over the trendy menu, offering drinks like "jade garden tea" and "honey lavender lattes." He asked me to order first and once I did, he simply said "make that two." It made us both laugh, which swept away some of the tension and what little awkwardness remained.

We found a booth at the back where it was thankfully quiet and empty. For the next four hours, we talked about everything and anything. Unfortunately, he didn't have any pictures to share (cuz, "flip phone"), but I did, and we proceeded to look through every photo of family that I could find—including the pets!

Dean shared stories of several family members. Each time he brought up a new name, we would use my phone to find them on Facebook. He would occasionally say, "you look like…" as we went through the various photos. Or he would say "you remind me of…" or "you're going to love…" as though he was confident this wouldn't be our one and only meeting.

It seemed difficult for him to hear about my mother giving me up for adoption, as well as other portions of my story. The parts that were the

hardest to live through were the parts that he clearly struggled with the most. What was most difficult for me to hear were the things he said about having some inclination that I existed. He told me that Cathy had told him she thought I might be his and that he met me once when I was a few weeks old. Immediately, the story she told about him holding me and saying I wasn't his came to mind.

He also told me that one of my mother's friends (he couldn't recall her name), called him once when I was a child to tell him she had seen me and that I was "definitely a Payne girl."

Perhaps one of the most shocking pieces of information he shared was that about 10 years ago, he told his now wife that, "There may be a knock on the door someday and it may be a woman saying she's my daughter." *That* piece of information sticks with me to this day.

Eventually, it got late enough that my husband, called to see what was going on. He was surprised to hear that Dean and I were still together. He was on his way home from work, driving right by the café and he really wanted to pop in. I asked Dean how he felt about meeting Tom and he was happy to oblige.

When Tom arrived the two of them shook hands and we all shuffled back into the booth. Dean and I relayed some of the day's events to Tom including the experience at the lab and how long it would take to get the DNA results back.

I could tell Dean was getting tired, so I told him I needed to get going. I got the feeling that he would've stayed there with me until they kicked us out if that's what I wanted him to do. We snapped one quick photo together before we left.

In the parking lot, Dean gave me a big hug and another kiss on the cheek. We stood there, awkwardly staring at each other for a moment,

both feeling the weight of our emotions-both with tears in our eyes. He was the first one to speak. "Thank you for today. This has been such a pleasure, babe." Then he paused, as though debating with himself. Finally, he took a deep breath and said…

"I really hope you're my daughter."

I couldn't speak. I could barely breathe. On the list of *"Things You Can Say to Heal a Heart,"* that was at the top of the list. I couldn't hold back the tears. Even as I write this, I can't hold them back. In the shakiest voice I eked out "Thank you. I really hope so too." And we embraced one more time.

As I started to walk away, he called out with a sheepish laugh, "So, what do we do now?!"

I turned to face him and shrugged with a smile, "I guess now we wait for results. Hopefully, it won't take that long."

"OK, but let's talk tomorrow. I will call you." He said it with certainty.

"Great! Looking forward to it. Drive safely!" And with that, Tom helped me hobble to my car. He opened my door and helped me in with a healthy dose of "I thought you weren't supposed to be driving." I barely heard him. My mind was busy playing over the events of the day. Especially those precious, last few words Dean had said before leaving.

Driving home, I was already looking forward to talking with Dean the next day. But the cautious, perhaps cynical part of me didn't want to believe that he would call. It was exhausting to hold back the hope, hold back the joy. Looking back, I wish I had been able to do a better job of holding all those emotions in tension with each other. But my father-wounds were still tender spots in my soul. My urge to self-protect was too strong to allow for that kind of vulnerability.

I wasn't on the road to home more than a few minutes when my phone rang. It was the hubs checking on me. "How are you doing, babe?"

"I'm OK." *Liar face.* "What did you think of him?" I asked with expectation.

"I think he's a really nice guy." He said sweetly. "And I think he's your father."

Too much. Too soon.

"I know you're trying to be encouraging, and you may be right. But BABE! I'm going to need you to NOT say things like that yet, OK? I'm not ready to get my hopes up and I'm not ready to believe he's the guy, let alone think about all that comes with finding him."

"OK. I get that. But I'm just telling you, *he's the guy."* And he said it with far more confidence than I was able to muster in the moment.

That night and the next couple of days were difficult. "Difficult." What a lame word to use for how the next few days felt. I literally prayed through each day of waiting for the results. I didn't sleep well. My appetite was fickle. My dreams were weird. My musings bordered on the irrational at times. In the span of 30 seconds I could believe without a shadow of a doubt that Dean was my father and in the next heartbeat I was completely convinced he wasn't.

Two dear friends, Andrew and Caitlin, our pastor and his wife came for a special visit. I say "special" because she was days away from giving birth to their first child, a daughter, Junia. And I was banking that Junia would be born on my birthday. (Spoiler Alert: *She was!)*

As I told Andrew and Caitlin the story, in true friend and pastoral form, they asked many good questions, but camped out on wanting to know

how I was feeling about everything and what they could do for me. Naturally, I asked for prayer. They were all too happy to oblige. My prayer request was a mix of maturity and little girl dreams. "Please pray that he's the one. Even if God has to bend the laws of biology to make it so" (a little girl's prayer), "Please pray that my heart and my family are protected in this and that God will work it out to His will and for His glory," (my more mature side).

Then, Caitlin so sweetly added, "And if he is her father, pray for lots of good health so they have the opportunity to make up for lost time." What a perfect and beautiful addition to our prayers.

We sat close on the comfy couches in our great room and brought the desires of our hearts to Jesus. There were tears and laughter and a sense that God was in that place. (Or, should I say "this place," as I'm writing this portion of the book from the very couch in the very room where we prayed those prayers.)

"When will you get the results?" Andrew asked.

"They said around five days, but they also said it could be sooner. Of course, I'm praying for sooner. My friend Julie seems to think I'm going to get the results on my birthday. Which would be crazy and awesome. Or *terrible* if he's not the guy."

"But it would be really cool if you got the results on your birthday and he is the guy!" Caitlin added.

True that, Caitlin. True that.

Generations/Family Relationships Chart reference, page 347

YOUR TURN: Reflect. Engage. Write.

My Dear Friend, How are you feeling about this portion of the story?

Does it remind you of anything in your story, of a time when perhaps you were hoping for something that seemed to hold the power to help you heal?

In this portion of my story, can you feel how I was wrestling with hope? It felt like a dangerous proposition, to lean into it. To trust it. Can you think of a time in your life when you wrestled with hope? When it felt dangerous to hope?

Based on what you've read up to this point, what portions of my story might this experience influence and how?

What generational patterns could be broken if Dean turned out to be my father?

What parental wound(s) does this have the potential to influence?

What is this stirring for you in your own story?

CHAPTER 16 The Best Gift

HAPPY BIRTHDAY TO ME

December 5th came and went with no results from the lab.

Thursday (my birthday) came. Still no word. It wasn't going to be much of an eventful day. Between my broken foot and my husband's company Christmas party that evening, there wasn't much space to plan anything else. But Julie decided it would be a good idea to grab some lunch together at one of our favorite Mexican restaurants.

We had a wonderful lunch with lots of laughter, revisiting my time with Dean and a little bit of her gently encouraging me that it was OK to believe he was "the guy" because she could "see it." She also convinced me to call the lab.

I waited until we got in the car to call, and wouldn't you know it, the technician who answered the phone was the same one who had taken our DNA samples. And she remembered me. Not only that, but she said

"Oh! Yes! I have your results right in front of me. Funny, I was just getting ready to call you."

Yeah, "funny."

She asked me if I wanted her to email me the results (was she serious?!) and I politely told her, "no thank you. I would like to come pick them up if possible."

Julie made a quick turnaround and pointed the car towards the lab. My stomach was flip flopping and I had to work diligently to control my breathing.

I had to get a grip. My heart was racing. I knew I had to decide I would be all right before we made it to the lab. Otherwise this would wreck me.

Decide. Right now, Gina. Decide that you'll trust God no matter what happens and no matter what disappointment you may face. It was the mantra I needed to adopt. It was the only way I could get through, no matter what the outcome, and still have my heart and soul intact. I repeated it to myself one last time, took a deep breath and exited the car to get our results.

I trust you, God. Please don't let me down.

The moment we entered the lobby I could tell our tech had been waiting for us to arrive. She practically leaped from her chair, manila folder in hand.

"Hi there!" She said with compassion and cheer in her voice. "I have your results right here."

I hobbled over to her desk and reached my hand for the envelope, shaking like a leaf in an autumn breeze.

"Sorry," I whispered. "I'm shaking like crazy. I don't know if I can open this." She extended one end of the long envelope to me but lingered in letting go of the other. I realized she was waiting for me to look her in the eye. I raised my gaze from the envelope to her sweet face. She locked eyes with me, and as if she knew what I had said to God, whispered, "It's going to be all right."

I just nodded, unable to respond with words. I opened the envelope and began reading. But the page was covered in mostly letters and numbers.

"What exactly am I looking at here?" I asked with confusion and no shortage of frustration.

I mean, seriously? Why couldn't the paper state it simply?! Like "Congratulations! You found the guy!" or, "I'm so sorry, he's not the guy." Instead, it read like lab data, requiring specialized education or at minimum, an interpreter.

Our patient tech leaned over and pointed to the bottom of the page. "Just look at this line here, honey."

I followed her finger to the bottom where I read...

> ***"The alleged father cannot be excluded as the biological father of the tested child. Based on analysis listed above, the probability of paternity is 99.999999999%."***

DEAN PAYNE! You *ARE* the father!

God had come through. ***BIG TIME!!***

I nearly crumbled. I was weeping openly at this point. I looked up to see that our amazing tech was crying too. As was Julie. And a woman

waiting to get blood drawn, who had figured out what was happening, was crying as well. It was an emotionally charged space to say the least.

I quickly moved to a chair to sit down before I fell. I kept staring at the page, afraid to take my eyes off it in the event the answer would change. Julie hugged me and gave me a good natured "I told you so." We laughed, and I admitted I didn't want to believe it could be true until we had the results. But the truth was, all that time waiting, I had worked tirelessly to silence the voice within me that already knew Dean was my father.

"Oh my gosh! He's got to be on pins and needles, same as me. I have to call him!"

I knew he was as eager as I was to get the results. We had spoken every evening on the phone since the day I met him. He had called me that morning to wish me a happy birthday. He also asked me if I thought today would be the day we got the results. He shared with me how much he was hoping it would be. "Because it's your birthday," he added.

I grabbed my cell and punched in his number. He answered at one and a half rings. "Helloooo..." he said in his typical, cheery, playful voice. "Hey there, I'm at the lab and just picked up our results."

"Oh my gosh," his voice was shaking. "Well, is it appropriate for you to call me dad?"

I could barely eek out the words. Words I had been longing to say since...well, since forever. ***"Yes, Dad. It is."***

I couldn't help but giggle through my flowing tears. "It's *very* appropriate."

"I couldn't be more thrilled, honey. I was hoping you would be my daughter." I could hear both joy and tears.

"I'm so glad it turned out this way. I suspected it would. I love you, Gina. I can't wait for the rest of the family to meet you. We have a lot of time to make up for." I savored every word he said, repeating them in my mind.

Dean and I spent just a couple more minutes on the phone. Then we both said we had people who were waiting for news of the results. We agreed to circle back later in the day and fill each other in on what our families had to say about it all. He would start with his wife, sons and siblings.

Quickly, I heard my internal voice personalizing Dean's list of characters; *"That's my stepmom, brothers, aunt and uncles. My FAMILY!"* It was all so beautiful, this long-held desire of mine being fulfilled.

Something was happening in the deepest parts of my heart. Hidden wounds of uncertainty and pain I had been carrying for so long began to heal at deeper levels than ever before. It was the mother (or should I say "father") of all emotionally corrective experiences. I was praising my heavenly Father for this amazing gift of an earthly father.

Family.

Before Dean (*my dad!*) and I ended our call, he asked me when I could come to the Lake to see him. "Soon!" I said quickly, "very soon." So, we made a tentative plan, exchanged all-too-natural "I love you's" one more time and hung up.

I had begun to make my calls to share the news when calls began streaming in from numbers I didn't recognize. Now, normally I don't answer calls if I don't know the number, but for some reason I felt like I needed to answer these. And I'm glad I did.

"Hi, Gina? This is your Aunt Sal. I'm so happy for you and my brother, honey. I can't wait to meet you. I love you already, babe."

"Hi Gina, this is your Uncle Dale. Welcome to the family. Your dad is so happy. I can't wait to meet you soon."

"Hi Gina, this is your Uncle Dave. We're so excited to find out about you. There's a family reunion this summer. Can you come?"

"Hi Gina, this is your cousin, Kelly. We're so excited to find out about you! Can you come to Christmas Eve at my house?"

Holy-oh-my-wow!

There's a Scripture that says, "God will restore the years that the locusts have eaten." Those words kept coming to mind with each and every phone call, with every sweet and welcoming voice. And with each call came greater healing and a deeper sense of belonging. My heart filled. My soul at peace. "Happy" would be an understatement. What I was feeling was pure *joy*.

(By the way, I said "yes" to Christmas Eve. And the family reunion.)

The days that followed were filled with tons of phone calls from family and friends. One of my favorite conversations was with Josie.

"Is this my *Aunt* Josie?" I said playfully. "It sure is! Is this my *niece?"* She replied with a warm chuckle. "It is!" I laughed, "and I can't thank you enough."

"Aww, thank you for letting me be a part of it. Now, is it OK if I tell my daughters?" She asked expectantly. But I think she already knew the answer.

"Oh my gosh! Of course you can! I can't wait to meet them!"

"I'm certain they will feel the same way! OK, I'm gonna give them a call. Let's talk soon."

Her daughters, Erika and Andrea, were among the first family members I met face to face, along with two of my other cousins, Sam and Phil. Little did I know that they had all been pulling a little recon of their own and stalking me on Facebook. The story goes that they were concerned they would all be "too much" for me, until they came upon a photo my husband snuck of me with a glass of red wine in one hand and a honey cigar in the other. (Don't judge. Besides, I didn't inhale.) Apparently, that was enough to give them confidence that I could handle whatever antics they had to bring.

The first meeting with my cousins was better than I could have imagined. Time flew by, and soon we were all commenting that it was as though we've always been together. That meeting was closely followed by Christmas Eve where I had the privilege to meet and connect with even more family.

As we left that night, my heart was so full. I wish I had better words to describe it for you. Even now, words fail me as I think back on how meaningful it was to be in that room, with my family, to feel their love and hear their joy over Dean and me finding each other. This room of smiling faces, all speaking my name with such warmth and acceptance, was a far cry from those rooms filled with family when I was a child, speaking my name in disapproving tones and somber faces. So much redemption. So much healing.

Just a few days later we celebrated our first Christmas with my Dad, stepmom, brothers, sister-in-law, nieces and nephew.

For all their arguing about letting me buy them presents, it was clear they had all worked hard to find things they thought Tom and I would love as well. Of course, when it came to my Dad, the gift of choice was

obvious: a framed copy of the photo Tom had snapped of us that first evening we were together in the café. (Even though my face was puffy from crying, it is one of my favorite photos to this day.)

As the tearing of paper and opening of boxes settled, my dad had one more gift to give. He reached under the Christmas tree and pulled out a small, carefully wrapped package. "This one is from me and from your Aunt Sal." He handed me the box, but not before I noticed tears welling up in his eyes.

I opened the box and my breath caught in my throat as I took in the beautiful, antique sight before me. "It was your *Nana's* ring, and we know she would've wanted you to have it." I couldn't say anything at first. My eyes stung with fresh tears. I took the ring from its plush, blue velvet cushion inside the box and slid it instinctively on my pinky. "I love it, Dad. Thank you so much." A tear rolled down his cheek as he took my hand in his and looking down at the ring, he said, "That's where your Nana always wore it too." I was overtaken by a strange mix of joy and sorrow. So. Much. Joy. Yet sorrow that I would never meet this strong woman whom I've been told would have loved me.

I'm confident I would have loved her, too.

YOUR TURN: Reflect. Engage. Write.

Dear Friend, as you read through this portion, I understand you might be thinking "How can she say, 'I love you'? How can they both be ready to say that to each other?"

The truth of the matter is that saying that to him and hearing him say it back felt as natural as breathing. Sure, it packed a huge, emotional punch to hear those words for the first time. And yes, there were questions that had yet to be answered (some that still remain).

But simultaneously, it felt like the most natural, normal thing to say and hear. It's difficult to explain. Sometimes, you have to decide how you are going to feel about something. And sometimes, you can't help how you feel. Still, there are other times when those two instances are in agreement. This was one of those times.

Why do you think I was ready to hear this from my dad and why do you think I was ready to say it in return?

Does this portion of the story make you think about any portions of your own story?

CHAPTER 17 He Can Be Trusted

SOMETIMES YOU JUST KNOW IT'S A GOD THING

As winter faded into spring and spring into early summer, we were able to spend more and more time at the Lake house which afforded us ample opportunities to spend quality time with my Dad and extended family members who lived close by. Each visit was overflowing with conversations, laughter and sometimes tears. All of us were trying to make up for lost time. Many of those visits remain fresh and vivid in my memory, but one stands out above them all.

My Uncle Don and Aunt Barb, along with my cousins Nicki and her kiddos joined my dad in coming to visit. There were the usual lake activities as lunch sizzled on the grill.

We spent a good deal of our time reminiscing about the last few months and the God-incidence (it's like a "coincidence," except God is responsible for it happening) of our home being right across the water from Dean. We had a chance to share the story of how the home came to

be ours and all the crazy circumstances that surrounded us purchasing the home.

"It was only 11 days from our first viewing to our first night sleeping in it!" I shared. Everyone marveled at the speed and smoothness at which inspections were performed and documents were signed. The swiftness of selling our former lake place, and the inexplicable occurrence of the seller taking our lower bid on the new house, merely because we could close immediately shocked everyone. Including our realtor. (The other bidder was only two weeks behind us at a significantly higher offer). Of course, I said it was because the house was *supposed* to be ours. And now, we *all* know why." I reached over and squeezed my father's hand.

"So, when was your first night in the house?" inquired my cousin, Nicki.

"June 22nd," I said. "The weather was amazing! It was unseasonably cool in the evenings and mornings that weekend. Absolutely gorgeous! The ride in our boat with what little we were bringing from the condo was sooo smooth! It was really..." I trailed off from my chatter as I noticed the look on my dad's face when he spun around and looked me right in the eyes, shock registered on his face.

Before I could ask what was the matter, he said softly, "When did you say you first stayed here?"

"Towards the end of June," I repeated. "The 22nd." Dean's face filled with emotion. "What's up, Dad? You OK?" I was getting a little concerned.

"Yes. I'm fine. It's just... well, remember I told you about that man and his wife who talked to me about God? Well, the 22nd is right around the time I said that prayer and accepted Jesus." His smile was so soft and warm, lighting up his entire face as tears made his eyes glisten.

I couldn't say much, but I didn't need to. I just smiled at my earthly father as I cried more tears of joy. And mixed with the joy of finding my dad, was the joy of finding that God was making it clear to me and everyone else that this happened in *His* timing. That *He* was the author of this beautiful story. He could, in fact, be trusted. Not because He gave me what I wanted. But because He is good. All the time.

In that moment, I had a privileged glimpse into the space where my earthly father and heavenly Father met. And in that moment, it was my heavenly Father who made Himself clear. "*Now* you understand the timing. He wasn't ready to be your father until he was ready to be *my child*."

YOUR TURN: Reflect. Engage. Write.

Dear Friend, as I write this, my eyes are once again brimming with tears. I don't think there will ever come a time when I relive that moment without the emotions hitting me hard. And I hope they always will. An encounter with our God such as that deserves to be felt, not merely retold.

What about you? Does this remind you of times in your life when God intervened? Or perhaps you have some inexplicable tale that normal reason can't satisfy?

Would you be willing to entertain the possibility that God was responsible for that?

PART FIVE
Healing Present and Past

CHAPTER 18

Unexpected Places of Healing

THE GOOD WITH THE BAD

Before we move on to the next section, we need to talk about something that's not quite as blissful as things have been up to this point in the story of me finding my father.

In full transparency, there are still times when I must comfort the little girl within me, times when she's insecure about her father's love, of his desire to spend time with her or to never leave. There are times when I must reason with the rebellious, wounded teenager within, who wants to demand to be heard, who sees no reason to hold back anything. And, there are times when I wrestle with the cynical adult in me who warns not to let my guard down completely, to trust only so far and to stop any kind words shared by my biological Dad from touching the deepest parts of my heart and soul.

I want to tread lightly here, because I don't ever want to minimize the amazing experience of meeting my Dad, or my family. And I don't want

to overshadow the precious gifts God gave me in that season of my life and has continued to give me since they all entered my world.

But it wouldn't be fair to you and it wouldn't be fair to me if I left it there. So, I will take a risk here, and give you the rest of the story. And I will trust you to be able to hold it all in tension with the beautiful things we've shared in this story up until now. I want to do this because as you explore your own story, and the stories of those who have gone before you, it will be important for you to be able to hold a variety of emotions and experiences in tension with one another.

Despite all the things that went well through the process of finding Dean, alongside the amazing "God-winks" that transpired, I had a lot of questions and a lot of moments that were painful. I'd like to say they subsided with knowing my father and talking things through, but many things he said gave me reason to question even more. And sometimes? I felt the pain of doubt and rejection. While I have felt those things less as time goes on and become more and more acquainted with who he is now, there are still times when I question, still times when I feel the pain.

As you already know, Dean admitted to me that he had an idea I was his, that he'd even been told by one of my biological mother's friends that she was convinced I was his—*"A Payne girl."* One of the deepest wounds came when he admitted that he had, in fact, held me, but still felt unsure that I was his. According to him, and in all fairness, according to my biological mother as well, Cathy was also unsure. So, while I'm not angry with him now, I can't help but wonder what would have been.

It's impossible to completely keep at bay the thoughts of how much he really believed I was or wasn't his. And if I'm not careful, I can let my questions and heartache run away with me. If I'm not staying aware and holding it all in tension, those questions, wounds, doubts can serve as bricks used to build a wall between me and Dean, and the rest of the

family. And while I would be "protected" to some degree, I would ultimately be missing out.

Admittedly, there are a lot of questions that remain unanswered for me. There's a good chance there will never be answers to those questions this side of heaven. And I'm learning to be OK with that. I guess in the end, it's a tradeoff. At the time of writing this, my dad is 72. While he is a warm and loving person, there are some places I don't think he can go emotionally—not in his own life, and not in mine. I know he has a great deal of regret for not being in my life as I was growing up. He struggles to hear the more difficult pieces from my story and likes to say things like, "But look how amazing you turned out," or "You have a really good life now." And he's right. I do! And at the same time, it doesn't minimize the impact of what I went through to get where I am now. And it doesn't change the fact that those traumas from early in my life were significant.

I'm also well aware that just because he's not ready (and may never be) to hear the more difficult portions of my story, that doesn't mean he's oblivious to them. And it doesn't mean that he's not fighting his own demons about it all. If ever I begin to doubt that, I can remind myself of all the things he's done and said to make it clear. Things like, "I have a lot to make up for" and "I'm sorry I wasn't there, but if I could've picked your husband, I would've picked Tom." If those "hints" are ever too subtle to convince me, I'll remind myself of the times he's come right out and told me how sorry he is and how much he regrets the way things happened.

I must rely on my heavenly Father's strength to process all of this and of course, *really* good therapy. Good therapy and a good God have taught me not to hate those pieces of me that struggle to trust and surrender—but rather, to thank them and integrate them. Yes, I said *"thank them."* You see, in each of their own dysfunctional ways, they're trying to protect me, to prevent any further hurt or disappointment. Good therapy has taught me to recognize this and a good God helps me to reassure those parts of me that their efforts are no longer needed, that we are

"OK" and that we can take care of ourselves. Even if that means taking risks and allowing a little pain to enter in now and again. For there can be no growth, no love and no change without it.

As for the really, *really* hard moments? Well, most days, forgiveness has been a "one and done" when it comes to my Dad. Sometimes though, when I connect new dots, or when I realize there was something that transpired that would've clearly been different had there been the presence of a father in my life? In those moments, I must choose forgiveness anew. Not to the exclusion of acknowledging the sorrow encountered along my journey, but as a part of my healing process. And it is a *process*. I choose to forgive because if I choose otherwise, I rob myself, my Dad and others in our family of the gift that God has placed before us. Besides, I know a little bit about growing and changing and holding out hope that your kids will forgive you and let you love them well.

Please don't misunderstand me. I had to go through the battle inside of me that the choice to forgive created. And it was a *battle*. So, my Dear Friend, if you're going through a struggle with forgiveness today, let me encourage you to *lean in*. The freedom it will bring you is worth the fight.

You may be thinking, "But Gina, you have *no idea* what I've suffered." And you know what? You're right. I absolutely do not. But, right here, right now, I want to tell you that I'm so sorry you went through it. Whatever "it" was or is. It breaks my heart that you've not only suffered, but that you've continued to carry the weight of it.

You know what else? Whether you're ready to believe it or not, it grieves the heart of God, too. If you're not ready to believe it, that's OK. There was a time I wasn't either. If you'd like to talk about that, I'm here. Seriously, check the back of the book. *I mean it.*

Know that whatever you've experienced, clinging to unforgiveness will only prolong *your* suffering. Not theirs. I know this firsthand. Forgiveness

is never about minimizing your pain or denying that wrongs were done to you. It isn't about invalidating your experience or the consequences in your life because of what happened. And it certainly isn't about letting the other person off the hook by pretending what they did wasn't wrong. I want to make this next point crystal clear:

*Forgiveness is **not** the same thing as reconciliation.*

You can forgive someone without opening up the opportunity for them to hurt you again. Even if they don't come out and ask for forgiveness; even if they're toxic and unsafe to be in a relationship with, you can still *forgive* them.

Why?

Because in large part, forgiveness is about setting you free. And you have the God-given right to be free, even if the other person never changes. Even if they never admit the exact nature of their wrongs against you. As much as that would be the right thing to do and an awesome asset to your healing, the fact is that you know what happened. Hopefully, you've told someone else whom you can trust and who will help you feel validated. If you haven't yet, please find someone like that.

OK, one last thing about forgiveness before we move on. Sometimes the person who hurt us has changed. Sometimes, they realize, at least in part, the gravity of their wrongs against us. Sometimes that person is willing to hear our hurts; to validate them without making excuses for their behavior. If such a person happens to be in your life, and you can see the changes are real and relevant, that they have become a healthier, safer person, may I encourage you to take the opportunity to be heard by them? And then take the opportunity to forgive. Then, little by little, if it proves to be a healthy thing for you, and if they have proven they can add something good to your life, work towards reconciliation. That would be the ultimate goal. That would be the ultimate victory.

Over the course of my life, I have been the wounded, and sadly, I have been the Wounder. Broken people tend to break people. While my brokenness was not an excuse, it certainly did perpetuate a pattern of destruction. I'm so grateful to God for the healing He has allowed me to experience. And I am so grateful for the forgiveness of those I wounded. Especially my kids. My kids know the door will always be open for them to tell me how something I have done has impacted them. I want them to know the generational cycle of secrecy, silence and unanswered questions ends here.

A TIMELY EXPERIENCE

At the time of writing this portion of the book, I have had yet another opportunity to experience a moment of healing. I was not sure how (or if) I was going to include this story, but at the urging of some wise friends, I decided to share— mostly because it is a tangible example of how we can break generations of shame and silence by speaking the truth and leaving evidence of the truth for coming generations.

In tandem with my own journey of writing this past week, I have been reading the memoir of Dr. Edith Eva Eger titled *The Choice*. Dr. Eger survived Auschwitz. I'm currently reading the portion of her memoir in which she shares her own deep struggle to find the willingness to face the flashbacks and aftermath of the trauma she suffered.

Dr. Eger reluctantly came to the realization that avoiding her feelings held the power to not only destroy her, but to harm her children, and perhaps even future generations. In her realization of this and her reflecting on the healing process, she made the profound statement that brought me to share my current situation with you.

In reference to her own journey of discovery and healing, Edith states:

"No one heals in a straight line."

It was under the weight of that statement that I realized it was important to include the events of this past week in this book. This past week, the "discovering" took a deep and dramatic dive when I had the privilege of sitting with my father and other beloved family members to learn even more about the generations before me.

Generations I never knew. Who never had the chance to know me.

It was a real time example of how far the consequences of our decisions can reach.

But unquestionably, the most profound moment came when these people who have become so precious to me in such a short time handed me the weighty "family history book" and asked me to *record my name in the book.*

Suddenly, the book's "weight" took on a whole new level of significance.

Rather than writing my married name alone, they also wanted me to record the name I was given at birth—the name that only belonged to me for a few short months before my mother placed me for adoption. (The first time.)

The moment was heavy with emotion and just when I thought I would be able to keep it together, my father turned to me and said, "Write your mother's name in there too, babe."

As I looked at our two names together on the page, my mother's and mine, it hit me that this was the first time in over half of a century that they appeared connected as mother and daughter. These two names, that were sealed away. Replaced by new names. New relationships. Roles altered.

And what hit me even harder was the fact that our names now appeared on the same page as my father's name—a record of the veil of shame and secrecy lifted. It was as though some long standing wrong had been made right, as the bold ink on the page declared to future generations:

Father. Mother. Daughter. *These names belong together.*

As I celebrated recording our names (along with my husband's name and the names of our children and grandchildren) into the family history book, for just a moment, I found a deep grief mixing in.

Grief for what was lost.

Grief for what I might have been protected from.

Grief for what could have been.

Grief for what was left undone.

Mixed in with all the healing that therapy and faith have brought into my life, and amidst these loving and welcoming new relationships, these wounds, these places to grieve surfaced—very real, and very worthy of recognition.

Although that day filled some places I did not realize were empty, the experience revealed areas of my heart that still need attention.

Some things that seemed settled were stirred, and some things stirred were settled.

How is that possible?

Because no one heals in a straight line.

And so, my friend, it will likely be true for your journey too.

As you discover and heal and grow, new wounds (or perhaps new facets of old ones) may surface. Do not be discouraged. Do not take this as a sign that you are not healing. Or that you are stuck. It is often a sign to the contrary.

Uncovering the places that still need attention can be a sign that you are *still* growing; that you are recognizing the impact certain events had on your life, and you are willing to do the deeper work. Sometimes what we learn about one event in our lives can shed more light on an area we did not know needed more attention. Most likely in the moment, we used all we had available to us to process through and go as far as we could then. When we uncover more, we can go further.

Now, having said all of that, let me introduce one caveat. If you *are* feeling stuck, if you find yourself in the same exact spot time and time again, or if you find you can't get through a certain portion of your story without feeling triggered or stuck, please find a qualified professional to help you. No matter what, be kind to yourself, regardless of how the road looks. Believe it will take you where you need to go.

For the rest of my journey, I am taking inspiration from folks like Dr. Eger, who did not begin her intentional journey to healing until she was a mother of three and entering her education in psychology. (Incidentally, she took her inspiration from a fellow survivor, Viktor Frankl.)

We all need someone to remind us that the path to healing is rarely linear, but it is always worth the trip.

THERE'S ALWAYS MORE TO THE STORY

I did my best to include the stories from my life that helped paint the picture of generational brokenness, along with the picture of redemption. We will explore a bit more of the "redemption" part in the next section and beyond, but for now, I realize you may be left with some questions at this point.

As for the questions you might have about my story, perhaps I didn't fully connect the dots in some places. Or maybe in others I left out chunks of the plot line. In many of those places, it's a matter of having little to no memory of what or how some events unfolded. Sometimes, to give you more detail, especially as it pertains to how any patterns repeated after me would require me to tell a story that isn't mine to tell.

I am not generalizing here to minimize or avoid talking about any of it. My goal is to protect others that might be harmed by public discussion of some of those events. Some of my choices and actions caused enough damage. I will not add to anyone's injuries or risk damaging the hard work that has been done to heal and repair relationships by putting those stories in print for public consumption.

And as for the generational patterns of my "new" family, well, I am still discovering those. I can already see some of the things that have repeated in the generations as well as the fallout they created. But I can also see beauty and a lot of love and the mark of the healthier generations left on this side of my family, and they are encouraging.

Before we close Part Five, I would like to share some helpful relational experiences from my life thus far which I pray will inspire hope and ultimately get you thinking about some moments from your own life that have provided you with hope and healing. Sometimes, those experiences are difficult to find. Sometimes they are seemingly small when they occur, but later we realize their impact was monumental, as was

true for me. But most of the time, we miss them because we haven't yet learned what they look like, or the power they hold.

I had spent a lot of time rehearsing the negative experiences in my life more than the positive ones—which, although unhealthy, sort of makes sense. Like other individuals who have experienced trauma, rehearsing those experiences that harmed us or caused us pain, is often an attempt to make sense of what happened.

One of the biggest problems with rehearsing our traumatic experiences is that, as I have said before, ***the story we tell ourselves most often becomes most true***. This particular "negative brand" of rehearsal eventually turns into value statements about ourselves. What we rehearse is what gets reinforced.

One of the biggest problems with rehearsing our traumatic experiences is that the story we tell ourselves most often becomes most true.

To be clear, there is a difference between rehearsing our traumas and giving voice to what needs to be heard. In my own journey, I told my story to therapists and others close to me as a means of working through what happened in the past, which was impacting my present, and consequently, my future. But there was intentionality and a limit to the amount of times I would replay what happened to me. Fortunately, I worked with professionals who knew the danger of letting me tell the same damaging stories over and over again.

So, to you I say, *if there are things in your story that you have not told to anyone, and if you are not ready to share your story with others (or even a professional), then consider writing about what has happened and letting it live on the page until you are ready to share it with a trusted friend and a counselor.* By the way, there is no time like the present.

There is powerful research on the efficacy of writing your story down. Just remember to give yourself permission to write freely. It does not have to be eloquent or even fluid. It can be bullet points, written as a story, a list of facts, a list of feelings, whatever you need it to be. Just remember to be honest, stay out of judgments about yourself, and walk away from it when it gets to be too much.

Then, when you are finished, if you have not already included them, take a shot at writing about some of the positive events in your story too, even if you have to start with what you might initially label as "trivial." (No judgment. Remember?)

Please don't leave this step out! Rehearsing only the negative can prevent us from recognizing and giving voice to the positive experiences. And the positives are extremely important because they carry a value statement about us as well—usually one that says something like "I'm valuable, worthy of love and acceptance and good things."

Acknowledging the good experiences is not for the purpose of minimizing or denying the hard things we have been through. It is for the purpose of reminding us that good things have happened, and they can happen again.

PART SIX

Emotionally Corrective Experiences

CHAPTER 19 Turning Toward Healing

WHAT HELPS US HEAL

Earlier in the book, I mentioned something called an *Emotionally Corrective Experience.* In short, ECEs are experiences that perform sort of like an antidote to the emotionally and relationally toxic experiences we have faced. Often, the experiences that wound us early in life are related to our inability to have healthy relationships later in life.

But ECEs, over time, give us an opportunity to experience healing. What I love most about this is that Emotionally Corrective Experiences are tangible examples of the gift of redemption. As we are wounded within the context of relationships, it is also within relationships that we have opportunities to experience what can help us heal.

As an example, there is no shortage of father-wounds in my story. However, in my adult years, I have experienced some *really* beautiful and profound moments with men who were father figures in my life, whether spoken or unspoken. Those beautiful moments were redemptive for me in that they offered healing for some of those early relational wounds.

The same has been true for experiences in healing some of my mother-wounds as well.

I give you all this background before diving into a few examples of my Emotionally Corrective Experiences because I want you to be intentional in thinking about your own experiences as you read through mine. There was a time when I wouldn't have been able to recognize an ECE if it jumped up and bit me on the proverbial nose. My defenses were simply too high. I lived in an almost constant state of alert. Always scanning for danger.

Some of my ECE's were simply too loud and too bright to ignore. Between them and some therapy, my heart learned to trust those experiences. The result was like salve on a wound.

I want you to learn to recognize *your* ECEs, pursue them, and perhaps even create some for yourself. These are the experiences that help us tell ourselves a different story—a healed and whole story. These are the experiences that help us *rewrite* the story of who we are meant to be.

As you read this next portion of the book, allow your mind to conjure up the scenes. Perhaps some scenes from your own life will appear as a result.

HEALING WOUNDS

Thirty years ago, if you had told me that today I would be a licensed therapist, writing this book, after graduating with a master's degree from a seminary, working with all kinds of people to help them find freedom and healing (in the Name of Jesus, nonetheless!), most likely I would have laughed in your face and told you to pass me another shot of tequila.

The reality of where I am on my journey today has much less to do with me than it has to do with God. I am a living, breathing, chatty testimony to the power of His grace, mercy and healing. While I have experienced a tremendous amount of help and healing from therapy, I believe that only God could have orchestrated the life I live today.

Along the way, He has used many relational experiences, or ECEs, to help me heal. But sometimes, people confuse Emotionally Corrective Experiences with Corrective Emotions. So, before we look at ECEs in detail, I think it is important to make the proper distinction.

As I've already introduced, an Emotionally Corrective Experience is just that; *emotionally corrective.* These are the experiences that sort of help us go back in our story and find places where something in us was wounded to the point that an unhealthy thought or feeling about ourselves resulted. Or perhaps some sort of unhealthy coping mechanism or way of behavior was born. Possibly both. In an Emotionally Corrective Experience, we *experience* something, relationally, that helps to heal those broken places, which over time changes our lenses, allowing us to think, feel, believe and act from a much healthier place. Additionally, they help us build hope and trust and, what is even more significant, help reduce our shame.

A *Corrective Emotion,* on the other hand, is an emotion we experience that *corrects* an unhealthy or unhelpful way of thinking, feeling, believing or acting. For example, if I take something that doesn't belong to me and I feel guilty as a result of it, there's a good chance that it will *correct* my behavior in that I will make restitution for the thing I took or, at a minimum, never do it again.

The distinction is important because in light of my own experience and the experiences of many clients, I don't believe we can open ourselves up to the work Corrective Emotions want to do in our lives unless we have had some Emotionally Corrective Experiences first. Those experiences help *correct* our *identity;* they are like a shield from shame. ECEs

are a way of healing old wounds (that might not feel so old). They help us believe we are worthy of love and created for a better, healthier and fuller life.

Without the salve that Emotionally Corrective Experiences provide, we run a great risk of seeing Corrective Emotions as confirming what is wrong with us. We experience the Corrective Emotion as a trigger to deep-seated shame and it can become a catalyst to even more destructive ideas, beliefs, feelings and behaviors. In short, we see them as threats; something we must protect ourselves from. We see them as something that confirms our reason to feel shame.

Without the salve that Emotionally Corrective Experiences provide, we run a great risk of seeing Corrective Emotions as confirming what is wrong with us.

Without the love and kindness, nurturing and light that Emotionally Corrective Experiences can offer, we are unable to see the difference between something we might have *done* that was a mistake versus our very existence being the mistake. Where the Corrective Emotion wants to tell us, *"You are better than this. Make a shift and try again,"* in the absence of Emotionally Corrective Experiences that have helped to heal some relational, and even some identity wounds, shame will twist the message. Instead, we will hear, *"See! There* ***is*** *something wrong with you! You are irrevocably damaged. Might as well continue screwing up. That's all you're capable of anyway."*

We need experiences inside of relationships, with others and with God, to remind us that we are not hopelessly broken or doomed to continue suffering the consequences of what's been done to us, or what we've done to ourselves (or even to others) as a result. We need to be reminded; to be shown examples that there is a better way, and that we are worthy and capable of finding it and living it out.

So, in the spirit of discovering those moments that have contributed to heath and healing, it is here that I would like to share a few of my own Emotionally Corrective Experiences.

DISCLAIMER: This list is *not* exhaustive. As I mentioned before, given the level of dysfunction I operated in for so long, it is highly likely that many more ECEs happened, but I was unable to recognize them. Perhaps they felt foreign, or maybe I did not trust them to be real and without ulterior motives. So, I did not let their impact sink in. But sometimes, ECEs are felt more implicitly and may not register cognitively. In other words, they can have an impact even if we do not readily recognize it at the time.

As I got older and began to actively pursue change and healing, the ECEs seemed to come more often. I can guess that was for several reasons. One, I was no longer content to allow toxic people to remain in my life. Two, I was learning to recognize when an ECE occurred, and three, I was finally willing to accept the work God wanted to do in my life. The biggest reasons have more to do with Divine intervention than anything of my own doing.

I hope you find the following examples from my story helpful. The goal in sharing them is to help you think about some ECEs from your own story that you might not have previously recognized as such.

Sister Debbie

When I was in second and third grade, there was this amazing teacher at the Catholic School I attended: *Sister Debbie*. She was so young! I remember thinking, "Wow! She's so fun and young! I can't believe she's a nun!" The rest of the nuns at my school where like drill sergeants on their best days, and prison wardens on their worst. But not Sister Debbie. She was kind and full of light and life.

She called out the best in me, and she did it with patience and compassion. She saw my love of all things art and fostered it every chance she got. I think she saw my pain, too.

Whether playing guitar, singing, drawing, and painting, or writing poems and stories, she championed my efforts. Most of the nuns treated me like I had the plague. Or that I was one. (If you recall, one nun warned a friend's parent to keep her daughter away from me because I was from a "broken home.") But not Sister Debbie. She gave me every opportunity to use my talents, explore my interests and expand them. She kept me focused on what I loved and encouraged my efforts.

She gave me a permanent spot in the guitar choir, allowed me to lead the school in worship songs during church and pulled me into every art project she created for the second and third grade hallways. She also let me write and put on a play for the entire second and third grade body.

Sister Debbie found ways to keep me close after school by asking me to help her with projects. I think she knew home was a dark place for me and that I didn't want to be there. She spoke life and light into my darkened world. I remember feeling the deepest sense of peace when I was around her—and a sense that she truly enjoyed my company, instead of seeing me as a burden.

My Biological Mom, Cathy

The details of this ECE are a bit fuzzy as I was half awake and half asleep, but I do remember much of it. She had built a room for me in the finished basement of their home, complete with trendy all-white furniture, adorned with colorful crystal drawer pulls. On the walls was large, neon floral-print wallpaper. By my childish standards, it was a pretty cool room.

I was already in bed and Cathy came down to chat with me. I sort of dozed off in the midst of our discussion, but I "half-woke" to her stroking my hair and telling me that she loved me and was going to make up for lost time with me. I suppose I could have opened my eyes but being not quite awake enhanced the magical dreaminess of what she was saying. It was the first time I remember feeling wanted by a parental figure.

I think more than anything, Cathy wanted a second chance at being my mom. As I'm sure you remember from earlier, her home with my stepdad wasn't any healthier than the one I was living in. But looking back I do believe she tried. And at this stage of my life I can say I love her for that.

Bill and Cindy

Bill and Cindy were the first people to ever pray over me. I don't mean ever pray over me there "at the church," I mean to *ever pray over me*. Yes, I was brought up in a religious home, and yes, we spent a lot of time at church. By that, I mean every weekday during my Catholic school career, on Sundays and every "Holy Day of Obligation." But, well... that doesn't make you any more of a Christ-like person than spending a bunch of time in a garage makes you a car.

I can't explain it, but something deep within me began to shift that day when Bill and Cindy prayed for me. There was no judgment or condemnation when I shared some of my struggles. There were no expectations or conditions set before me—just praying over me and inviting me to their home for prayer and Bible study. They were some of the first people who ever showed me the real Jesus and I think they are part of the reason I eventually came around to believing in His great love and mercy for me.

Tom

My first ECE with my husband was an important shift in recognizing that a healthy relationship was possible and that I was worthy of being heard. We hadn't been dating long, and while I don't recall the exact circumstances of the conversation, the important part that sticks with me is how he handled me telling him that he had hurt my feelings by what he had done and said. From the time I was a child, I remember being responsible for how everyone around me felt. I learned at a young age that if I was sad or afraid or anxious or whatever, it was my problem and it was most likely due to something I did or didn't do.

Consequently, just telling him how I felt was an enormous risk on my part. In previous relationships, that had been proven a very unsafe thing to do either physically or emotionally. And, since our brain reacts the same to a physical threat as it does an emotional or perceived threat, my mode of self-protection became to shut down and shut off to avoid getting hurt in any and all circumstances.

But for some reason, that day something was different. I took the risk and I told Tom that what he had said and done really hurt my feelings. The details of his response remain vivid, because the emotions that were attached to the experience were so strong. That is called "emotional salience." That's why all of your most vivid memories have very strong emotions attached to them.

I clearly remember saying the words, "That really hurt my feelings." And then holding my breath.

He was silent for at least 12 minutes (just kidding). Tom's reply was short and to the point: "I'm sorry, babe. That was not my intention, but I can see why it would upset you."

While his answer was not wordy or full of deep emotional contemplation, it was everything I needed to hear. What he said was that he was sorry and could see my point of view, what I *heard* was "your feelings matter and the way you see things matter and I want you to know that you matter to me." The freedom to be me in our relationship was handed to me in that moment. I believed the possibility of better-than-what-I-had-known was not only possible. It was a reality. He continues to prove that to me every day.

Another Debbie

Right after Tom and I were married, I felt a pull on my heart to leave my job and to be more available to the kids. I had begun attending a new church and with it came a pull to get involved with helping people. I knew I wanted to work with women who were fleeing abuse or struggling with homelessness or any other identity-robbing, freedom sucking situation they might be in. I knew firsthand the anguish of such situations, and I longed to help others experience the kind of shift I had experienced.

So, at a little church in Ellisville, Missouri, I met a woman who became sort of a "spiritual mama" to me (she would be the first of two amazing women to fill that role in my life). The irony of her name being *Debbie* was not lost on me.

We were working through a book together to help me deepen my faith and to grasp what it meant to become a more intentional follower of Jesus. This was me searching, no one was persuading me—other than the Holy Spirit.

Deb was patient and kind. She prayed for me all the time (and still does), and never put any heavy burdens or expectations on me. But one of the most important gifts she gave me was her belief in me. She never

seemed to consider my past as an obstacle or sign that I couldn't "cut it" as a believer. She never treated me as damaged or disqualified. She was an echo of my first, precious ECE, Sister Debbie.

We met weekly, at the little church office. On this particular day I arrived fresh from having just watched a show in which the host asked everyone in the audience what they would do to help others if they knew they could not fail.

"What would you do if you had one hundred dollars and wanted to make a difference in this world?" she said in her best announcer voice. After interviewing some incredible people who had built whole organizations to help people in need, starting with just one hundred dollars, the host then proceeded to give everyone in the audience a hundred-dollar bill to go out and start doing. I thought that was such an inspired idea! The stories were too incredible to keep to myself and I couldn't wait to share them with Deb.

"Wow!" she said. "That's amazing!" Then she paused and tilted her head to the side, offering up an equally tilted smile as she often did before posing a deep question. "I'm curious, what would *you* do with one hundred dollars if you believed you could not fail?"

The answer poured out of me like it had been dammed up for centuries. "I would help women who are hurting, like women who are homeless or in dangerous home situations—maybe even single moms who are struggling and need help. You know, women who've had a hard life. Women who don't have family to turn to. I'd help women like me—er—like I was."

The next thing I knew, she was encouraging me to tell the story to the rest of the church "You never know," she said. "God just might be up to something."

And it was there that my first ministry was born—one that would see many women and children walk through our doors to find resources, hope and healing. It happened because of the encounter God orchestrated with Deb—because she believed in me. It didn't occur to her to think I couldn't do it, or that I shouldn't.

And it was because of that church and that little ministry that I met two of the most precious people in my life, Chrissy and Julie. Over the past 20 years, Chrissy and Julie have been my "emotionally corrective experiences" in more ways than I can count. I consider them two of my brightest symbols of how God restores the years the locusts have eaten.

Later in life, God would see fit to bless me with a heaping handful of unique and precious friendships that I can say have each contributed in some way to my healing and growth. I am grateful for and love each and every one of them.

You already know about some of the experiences with my biological dad and how healing they were, but there were men along the way in my adult life who also provided some healing in the area of fatherlessness.

Simon and Dan

It was towards the end of my internship year in grad school. Our fearless, rag tag group of seven soon-to-be-therapists had been through the trenches with each other. We had shared our genograms (the stories of how we came to be us as influenced by familial generations past, and by past and present relationships). We had supported one another through difficult personal experiences over the past few years, and in particular through that last year. We celebrated with one another and offered encouragement and on rare occasions, advice when it was asked for. We dove in deep with our hearts and souls.

During one Friday's supervision session, we were sharing how it was going at our respective counseling sites. Each of us had been assigned a specified counseling center in which to see clients and satisfied our internship hours requirement. While I was already over the required hours, I was still at both of my sites. One was going extremely well. The other?

Not so much.

I was recounting one of the more frustrating experiences with my site supervisor that had hit me deeply. I was feeling the kind of soul-tired you feel from caring for others in an environment that is void of support or encouragement for the work you are doing. I had shared the details of the experience which was met with many nodding heads and sympathetic looks from my group.

When I was finished, our professor, Dan, offered some sort of quick response that felt very dismissive (which was highly unlike him) and went on to the next person in the group who had something they wanted to share. As that person began to speak, Simon gently interrupted them. "Sorry to interrupt you," he said with a hand up in front of him. Then turning to me, he said "Gina, did you get what you needed from us just now in response to what you shared?"

Tears stung my eyes. My face felt hot and I struggled to make eye contact. It was the moment of truth. I felt more seen than I had in a long time and the shock of it was like plunging into ice cold water on a hot summer day. Except this *wasn't* cold. It was warm. So. Warm. And loving.

"Thank you, Simon. And actually, no. I didn't." Each face reflected compassion and care. Including our professor's. "OK, thank you." Simon said. "Would you tell us how we missed the mark for you?"

Dear Friend, can you see how Simon's words, all on their own, were incredibly corrective for me? I am not sure I could recall a time when someone asked me that question. *"How did I miss the mark?"* What I heard in that was, *"How did we not see, hear, know you the way you needed to be seen, heard and known. How did we not love you well?"*

I couldn't recall a time or a place when I would've felt safer to reply honestly to such a question (other than with my husband).

I was able to share with the entire group how dismissed I felt by my site supervisor and how frustrated I was not having someone to celebrate a client's breakthrough with after the long road I'd walked with them. I shared how defeated I felt when my site supervisor didn't approve of my methods, and how confusing that was given how careful I had been with this client and how I implemented exactly what I was learning.

I even shared how it triggered so many instances in my life when an authority figure told me, whether implicitly or explicitly, that I wasn't enough. I found myself crying in the middle of the group with six other faces looking at me with compassion. Each took their turn sharing what they heard in my story and how frustrated they were with my site supervisor. They helped me feel validated and affirmed in the work I was doing as a therapist with my client, but more importantly, as a person.

Then came Dan's turn to respond. "I'm sorry I didn't offer more when you shared your experience, Gina. The truth is that I was too busy trying to hide my frustration with the way your site supervisor handled the situation. You deserve more than that. You're doing good work with that client and you deserve to be supported. I'm also aware that this isn't the first time you've had a difficult experience there.

"And I think at this point, I'm going to release you from your site and let your supervisor there know why. It's not OK. And I'm sorry this happened. And I'm sorry I didn't protect you from it sooner. You deserve better."

Simon smiled at me and said, "How are you now?"

"I'm better," I said with a sigh. Pausing to let it all sink in deeper I replied, "Actually, I'm good. Thanks, Simon."

But for me, it wasn't over.

Thankfully, group supervision was the last class of the day on Fridays. Afterwards, I hopped in my car and headed for home. I was on the road for all of about five minutes when the events of what transpired in group came back, replaying like a movie before my eyes.

The realization that the words spoken over me by Dan had never been uttered before, hit me with a tidal wave of emotions. It was the first time I could remember when a male authority figure in my life said he wanted to protect me. There were no ulterior motives in his concern. It was this simple: *he cared that I had been hurt and wanted to do something about it.*

I didn't need to earn that from him. I mattered. My feelings mattered. He wanted to champion me in my experience with my site. He wasn't just defending the way I was counseling, he was defending *who* I was at my core. Because ultimately, that's where you counsel from in the first place.

Before that day in group, I can say in all sincerity that I couldn't recall a single experience where I communicated an emotional need to someone in authority over me and had that need met. You know how when you pour water on cracked and dry soil, the water quenches the soil's thirst and fills in all those little cracks and crevasses, making the ground whole again? Well, Dan's words and actions found some of those cracks and crevasses in me that day and filled them in.

Learning

There were times when corrective experiences were more intrinsic, like what God showed me during graduate school. But throughout the course of my time there, I had many opportunities to learn more about myself, my wounds, and the wounds of my mother(s) in my class work. I also learned more about a disorder I mentioned earlier, Borderline Personality Disorder. I realized that Cathy exhibited traits of this disorder. Those traits presented behaviorally in Judy, Julie and from what I understand, in Marie as well. This made a lot of sense to me given the thread that inextricably connected their lives.

Most of these revelations came when we were required to read a specific text called *Understanding the Borderline Mother.* I found myself swept away as the words on its pages described much of my experience with the female caregivers in my family. Reading the book was a mix of relief, anger, grief and compassion. I was relieved to find further evidence that I was not crazy, and angry that this information was not brought to light for my mother(s) when I was growing up. I felt grief for what might have been, along with compassion for what they must have been experiencing mentally and emotionally, with no one to help them and no means of understanding what must have felt dark and hopeless. Learning about BPD at a deeper level offered me a tremendous amount of freedom and clear direction on how to proceed even deeper in my own therapy. In light of that new information, with the help of a therapist, I was able to reframe so many events from my childhood, attributing the gravity of my experiences in part to this undiagnosed disorder. These women in my life, while still responsible for their behaviors, were *suffering*. Consequently, I was suffering too. In knowing this, my compassion for them and for myself deepened.

The healthier we become, the more the lenses through which we see the world, and other people (including our past) begin to adjust. We see things in a different light than we once did. We begin to recognize

those spots that were like an oasis in the desert that was our life. Those moments of learning and realization can be ECEs in and of themselves.

Before we end this section, I want to share one more ECE in my life— Admittedly, there is sorrow mixed in with the experience, but it's simply too big of a God-encounter to not include. So, here we go…

Michael

I told you that I was blessed with an incredible group of people in my internship year and cohort group, but there was one person in my group with whom I had a connection deeper than either of us knew.

In 2015, the oldest of my half-brothers on my mother's (Cathy) side, Dave, reached out to me with a very sweet, very apologetic message asking if I would like to talk. It had been 18 years since we spoke, 18 years since I spoke with anyone in my biological mother's family.

The message was somewhat disorienting. I listened to it over and over to see if I could hear a different message than the one he was *actually* saying. But I didn't. He was sincere. So, I left him a message back. Eventually, we agreed to meet. I was apprehensive but also excited to know his three children whom I had never met—two daughters and a son— my nieces and nephew, Maddy, Savannah-Rose and Gabe.

In his messages, Dave said he wanted to make sure I knew that Cathy had died the year before, and that our brother, Christopher, had died months before her. Cathy died on Mother's Day. This was difficult news to hear—news that threw me back into therapy for a while, for all the reasons you might expect and for a few you might not.

Seeing Dave face to face was an incredibly emotional reunion. I got the chance to tell him the story of me that he never knew, including my

uncle's attempted assault and the pain I experienced from David, his own father. He told me how difficult his own relationship had been with his father as well, and that they had been estranged for quite some time. None of this was a surprise.

Then, I got the opportunity to meet his kids. It was a sweet time of learning about them and answering a million of their questions about me and my family. They pulled out all the photo albums and I pulled out the photos on my phone. We laughed a lot, cried a little and bonded through all of it.

I decided to take them all out for dinner and the kids wanted to ride in my car. We had a blast on the short jaunt to the restaurant, laughing and lovingly teasing each other about all kinds of things, family resemblances, funny habits, current crushes.

The two older children allowed the youngest, Savannah (Rose for short), to sit in the front which was so kind. At one point, she leaned over and whispered in my ear "Hey Aunt Gina, ask Maddie about Matt *(last name removed for privacy)*." I froze in my seat. *I knew that name.*

Savannah chattered on as Maddy's face turned red as she giggled in the back seat.

"He's a boy at our church. His dad is kind of a pastor or counselor or something. Maddy has a BIIIIIG crush on Matt." She beamed a smile back at her big sister.

"Is his dad's name Michael. Er, Mike?"

"Yep!" Maddy said. Then, she leaned forward, "Aunt Gina, do you know him?!"

"Yes," I choked out, fighting back tears that threatened to spill, "I believe I do."

Mike had been a dear friend and member of my cohort group in grad school. I couldn't wait to call him after dinner. When I was finally able to reach him, I was shocked to hear just how deep our connection went. He not only knew my family, but he and his wife (coincidentally named Gina) had been "doing life" (a Christian vernacular for walking with someone through the tough things in life) with Cathy and David before she died. I needed to know more, and so did he. So, we met for breakfast.

"I can't believe I didn't make the connection." Mike had listened to me tell most of my story in our cohort group. He knew my biological mother's story too. But he never connected the dots.

"Remember that week when I was late to cohort because I was visiting a woman from my church in the hospital down the street? That was your *mom!*" I watched as tears accumulated in his eyes. "She was in the hospital with complications from her diabetes."

"Ultimately what she died from," I added in a whisper.

The gravity of what he revealed hit me immediately. Mike was literally in the presence of my mother and me *on the same day*, multiple times. Every day for three and a half years, Mike and I walked through our counseling program together. All the while he was walking through life with my mother. Yet the two worlds never collided.

"I can tell you this though, your mother died knowing Jesus. She was absolutely a follower of Christ. And she loved you, too. Granted, I didn't know it was *you*, but she did love 'her daughter.' You *will* see her again one day, my friend." He struggled to get the words out, emotion thick in his voice.

I will see her again one day.

Mike and his wife had helped Cathy find some healing on this side of heaven. They were walking with her to help her grow in faith and emotional wellness.

Mike was also present, walking with me as God used the counseling program to help me grow and heal, too. He was an important part of my support system, and I was a part of his. But on this side of heaven, for whatever reason, God did not see fit to bring my biological mother and I together on the journey. Instead, he connected us through Mike, for the time when I was ready to hear about her.

I take the whole experience to be an example of God's protection over me and perhaps, over Cathy, too. This was the way it had to be. But not forever. Because of what Mike knew and shared, I know that someday I will see her again. And in that moment, all will be more than forgiven. It will be forgotten. Not in a Pollyanna sort of way. But in the most profound way imaginable. We will both be new, fully restored. Fully healed. For me, somehow, the knowledge of this resolves all the unsaid and all the undone between us. In this moment, I can say with confidence that she is experiencing the same thing, too. Reflecting on that truth is an emotionally corrective experience all to itself.

Me

I believe this particular ECE is one you will find encouraging. It is an ECE I had with *myself*. During the time of writing this, we are in the throes of a pandemic. To fight the isolation required to prevent the spread of the virus, people are looking for creative ways to engage without putting themselves or others at risk.

In my neighborhood, this has taken the form of things like scavenger hunts, homes putting up holiday lights early for families to come by and enjoy, hearts in windows with positive messages, and my personal favorite, painted rocks.

So, I decided to paint a variety of rocks to place around the neighborhood, then announced it on the neighborhood's Facebook page, and offered prizes for the first to find a rock, snap a photo and post. I was pleased with how much joy this simple thing brought to our little community.

One particular evening, as I was creating rocks for another round of find-and-post, I took a break from painting to load the dishwasher.

I was feeling happy about my project when suddenly, anxiety hit. This little voice from within kept prodding me to "hurry up" and load the dishwasher. This voice was followed by internal messages like "you're wasting your time on those rocks," and "you need to hurry up and get things done that matter." I chose not to entertain the message and instead, decided to get *curious* about it (a powerful weapon in the pursuit of growth). I got quiet, shot up an arrow prayer, and asked God to help me figure out *"who does this message sound like?"*

There was no one person that came to mind. Instead, multiple memories came to mind of times in my earlier years when I felt like an inconvenience to the adults in my life. Times when the message of "hurry up" was barked in my direction because I was taking too long to get ready, to learn something, to eat, even to go to the bathroom. If I didn't hurry, there were always consequences.

In that moment at the dishwasher, the little girl in me was trying to get me (us) to hurry up so that we would "be OK." Rather than acquiesce, I chose I different route.

"We're OK. AND—We do not need to hurry."

I could *feel* the shift. My shoulders released. My stomach calmed. Peace entered. The lie the little girl in me believed (and had carried for so long), was revealed for the falsehood it was. With God's help, *I* was my own Emotionally Corrective Experience.

I share this particular ECE because I believe it's important to recognize your power here, to learn to create these experiences for yourself. God has equipped us for this. While sometimes He provides the ECE Himself; other times He empowers us to make it happen. And often, He empowers us to help others experience them, too.

I hope to have many more ECEs in my life. Each one a reinforcer of God's presence and provision for me. Each one bringing me deeper into who I am called to be and into my purpose in this world.

NOTE: I want to be clear that, while I did not have a separate entry for Jesus in my list of Emotionally Corrective Experiences, the reality is that He gets the credit for all of them. It shouldn't go without mentioning that every person in my list was/is a believer in God and a follower of Jesus. I realize that won't be the case for everyone who reads this. However, whether you can easily see it or not, and I would go so far as to say, even if you're not sure you believe it, every good thing that helps us heal is a gift from the Creator of all good things. If you haven't given Him a chance to work in your story, consider this an encouragement and invitation to do so now.

YOUR TURN: Reflect. Engage. Write.

Dear Friend, as you read through my personal examples of Emotionally Corrective Experiences, I hope you have been able to see them for the powerful force they are. Remembering moments like these are important, even if you have the darkest of pasts. These moments are the most valuable of treasures. I would argue that the harder your story has been, the more important finding your ECEs becomes.

Maybe your ECEs were instances when someone did or said something that gave you reason to believe in yourself, or reason to believe that there are good people in the world who will love you and champion you.

Maybe someone introduced you to a talent you have or taught you about a sport or subject that you absolutely love, even to this day. Perhaps someone helped you feel seen and heard, they accepted you just as you are.

Right now, take some time to set this book aside and write down as much as you can about your own ECEs. If you can clearly see the connection between those moments and something good in your life today, (like I did with Sister Debbie encouraging my writing) then please make sure to write that down, too. This will prove to be a powerful exercise worth doing.

And just in case you are *really* struggling to come up with an instance from your past, let me offer one in your present. Hear my words: *You, my Dear Friend, are an incredible person. Yes, you. No matter what you've done, no matter what has been done to you, Beautiful Soul, you are of great worth. You are loved. Deeply. You are braver than you know. The fact that you are reading this book and examining your own story proves it. I see you, I believe in you and I am cheering you on.*

PART SEVEN

Jesus and A Therapist

CHAPTER 20

Mental Health in Christian Circles

THE CASE FOR HOLISTIC HEALING

Throughout our time together, you have heard me mention the importance of both Jesus *and* a therapist. So, I hope it feels like a natural progression to now visit the value of having both present in your healing journey. I want to explore this more in depth and intentionally discuss how the two fit together—well, at least, how they have fit together for me, for countless friends, colleagues and clients. I want to draw attention to the importance of having both a relationship with God *and* a therapist because I have watched mental health handled poorly in some Christian settings.

Notice I said "some." Not "all." In fact, I know many qualified, clinically trained, Christian therapists and psychologists who have a healthy perspective and approach to mental health. I lock arms with them and champion them in their efforts. But this chapter is not about them.

This portion of the book is about shining a light on ideas that cause more harm than good "in the name of Jesus" and it has to stop. It is my hope

that in talking about it, we can bring awareness, so we can respectfully call it out when we see it. When we know better, we can do better.

Right out of the gate and as gently as possible, I want to call attention to a fact that is unpopular in some Christian circles: *people can heal from trauma and break unhealthy patterns of behaviors and beliefs outside of a relationship with Jesus.* Stick with me here...

There are therapists out there doing good work with those who are hurting and helping them heal from the pain of their traumas. Those caring souls are using evidence-based therapies to help people break free from wounds and change how they see the world and themselves.

While those practitioners may never utter the name of Jesus in their therapy room (or believe in Him at all), there is a common grace, granted by God, at work and present in the healing journey of the individuals they help. Common grace allows the sun to shine and the rain to fall on us all, regardless of what we believe. It is that same common grace that allows evidence-based therapies (including medication) to work for many people, no matter what they believe.

Those therapies work because they honor how we are created, how our brains are wired and how our emotions work. Whether explicitly mentioned or not, they align with how we are designed to be connected in healthy relationships, as we are created in the image of God who displays the ultimate healthy relationship between Father, Son and Spirit. Those therapies work because they are consistent with how God has designed us, whether they acknowledge Him as Creator or not.

So, if we want people to believe us when we say there is a whole other level of freedom *beyond* what they can experience through clinical therapy alone, and if we want to help people see that the deepest healing comes when we do that good, hard work within the context of a relationship with Jesus, then we must recognize and be respectful of the

benefits therapy provides, much like we would for people who are seeking proven clinical treatment(s) for their physical ailments or diseases (we would never tell someone that a relationship with Jesus alone is the answer to their cancer, or heart condition, or diabetes).

We must stop putting people in a position to feel they have to choose between Jesus and a therapist, or between Jesus and medication. We must end the twisted idea that people struggle with mental illness or the effects of trauma because "their faith isn't big enough." And we must give people in the church (whether sitting in the seats or standing on the pulpit) the freedom to speak openly about their journeys to healing when they include clinical interventions and/or medications, instead of expecting them to over-spiritualize their healing. That just peddles false hope and perpetuates shame. That isn't the way of Jesus.

As we wrestle with the idea of getting comfortable with people admitting that therapy, even therapy that may not overtly call on God, can be effective, here is something I want us to consider. Given the dynamics of some people's traumatic experiences, God may somehow seem to have been made culpable or complicit in their wounding. Perhaps the abuse or trauma they experienced was at the hands of a self-professing Christian. Or maybe they prayed for God to stop their abuse when it was happening. It could even be that an abuse was perpetrated in the name of Jesus or as punishment for not doing what God said they should do.

Many have prayed and prayed for healing or rescue, but no rescue or healing came. Maybe they have cried out to God to help them remember what happened to them or cried out to Him to stop the memories from flooding them. In any of those cases, if prayers went unanswered, it is likely they are not going to seek out God's involvement or trust God enough to allow Him to play a role in their healing. We must make space for them to travel the road to heal the way they need to. God can be the orchestrator of their healing even if they aren't calling on His

name. (Think "book of Esther" in the Old Testament. God was all over it, yet never mentioned by name.)

To try and force Jesus on someone might cause more damage and push him or her further from God. We must be willing to consider that perhaps God is using therapy to free that person up enough to learn to trust Him. Some who enter counseling may need to live in the freedom they find through therapy for a while in order to recognize that something is still missing. Therapy might be the very thing that allows them to open themselves up to trusting that God is for them. I can say that with confidence because that was me. And it has been true for a lot of my clients as well.

Therapists who practice from a redemptive worldview will honor where their client is and work in clinical ways that meet those needs. They will prayerfully discern when to bring Jesus into the mix as their client is ready. They recognize the importance of the spiritual side of our being, even if they are not trying to get us to label it. Look for those therapists. I promise you they exist. I personally know many. (I will even help you with a referral!)

STRUGGLING DESPITE OUR FAITH

And then, there is the proverbial elephant in the Christian room that no one really wants to talk about...

There are people who hold a firm and healthy faith in Jesus yet still struggle with a diagnosis of mental illness like anxiety, depression, schizophrenia, bipolar disorder and even PTSD, as well as a whole host of other challenges that are *not* the result of their sin, lack-luster prayer life or shallow belief. And the truth is they may never be completely free from their mental illness this side of heaven.

In thinking about those who fit that description, I include some in church leadership as well as those in attendance. Yet, many do not feel safe enough to be open and vulnerable with their struggles (especially those in leadership) for fear of judgment or their faith being called into question. They suffer silently in shame and pain.

There are a lot of hurtful ideas floating around out there that perpetuate the shame/pain cycle in Christian circles. One of my least favorites is "Jesus plus nothing." I literally wince when I hear it in Christian teaching or see it emblazoned on some kitschy meme on social media. I cannot help but think of all the people who love Jesus with their whole heart, mind and soul, but struggle despite their fervent prayers and unshakeable faith. My heart breaks to think a statement like this might drive them further into silent suffering, never allowing the light to touch their pain. Not understanding that sometimes, *The Light* can shine through a therapist.

"Jesus plus nothing," fits when it comes to the supernatural salvation and freedom we get to experience for all eternity. But when it comes to issues of mental health, "Jesus plus nothing" is not always the answer. Besides, we would not encourage people to pursue "Jesus plus nothing" for their physical illness.

Now, having said all of that, I want to make sure I do not leave out a very real, very important truth: *God can and does absolutely heal people, but that doesn't mean He absolutely will for every person and in every way.*

Yep. I said it. Because it is true. Even the Apostle Paul (undeniably a pillar of the Christian faith) who prayed for his "thorn in the flesh" to be taken away, ultimately did not receive that healing here on Earth. While sometimes God heals suffering, other times He *engages* with it instead. But we do not get to decide when He will do that, and we cannot take a formulaic, absolute approach to how either of those things will happen.

CHANGING OUR THOUGHTS

Still, we have many Christian teachers and, admittedly, even some therapists, who say we need *only* "change our thoughts" in order to "change our lives." (Which is ironic, because technically, that would be a *cognitive* approach. Not a *spiritual* one.)

And, in some ways, they are correct. Changing our thoughts has scriptural backing and a significant amount of science that agrees as well. It is in fact, a wonderful contributor to our healing and growth, with high relevance when discussing how we can improve our overall quality of life.

In fact, changing the way we think about things is one of the most powerful, life-altering activities we can engage in. We know the brain can learn to rewire itself, and we understand that many of our battles are fought in the mind.

But y'all! Even changing your thoughts is not a battle fought *just* in the mind! For whole healing, we need to consider our whole being. Jesus did.

He helped heal a woman's shame and the internal wounds of abuse by writing in the sand (John 8:1-30); He engaged in loving conversation with someone whom others refused to see (John 4:1-26); and He used the smell of fish over a fire as He cooked a little breakfast, paired with a heart to heart talk to heal a broken relationship (John 21:8-16).

If we are paying attention, we can see so many ways in which Jesus met the needs of the hurting, including speaking out and standing up for those in the throes of shame and humiliation, of those struggling mentally and physically and those who were spiritually abused and bullied. With each of these there was an interaction. A process.

Often, it is in the *process* of healing that God does the most work within us. What we glean and how we grow in the journey is often as powerful as the healing itself. It is what builds our empathy and compassion. It strengthens our wings and prepares us for flight. Our willingness to take the journey is, in part, what offers tremendous hope and encouragement to others still fighting for their healing or the healing of their loved ones.

For myself and countless others who recognize the need for professional help in their journeys, in *addition* to their relationship with God, let me say this: *Jesus takes it a step further, taking us where therapy alone cannot. His Divine presence in our story takes us from a place of healing to a place of redemption.*

Jesus takes it a step further, taking us where therapy alone cannot. His Divine presence in our story takes us from a place of healing to a place of redemption.

For me, His intervention allowed me to forgive at a level rarely achieved outside of relying on something greater than ourselves to help us carry it out.

Therapy helped me see that many of the unhealthy patterns in my life were not the result of my own creating. Those behaviors and beliefs went much further back than my years on this planet. Therapy taught me that my early life environment had been steeped in those unhealthy beliefs and behaviors which were *generations deep*, making it was almost certain that they would infect me as well.

Therapy is what helped me uncover emotions that could not be processed through mere talking or simply working to change my mind. It is what helped me release emotions that were sort of "stuck" in my body, something that in all likelihood would've never been achieved if I had simply stayed "in my head."

Therapy helped me see that there were parts of myself I had learned to hate and disconnect from, and, ironically, those were the parts that, when integrated into my sense of self and cared for well, offered some of my most significant healing.

Therapy provided corrective lenses to help me see so many things clearly, including my faulty thinking behind how I viewed God for much of my life as well.

I cannot imagine where I would be without therapy and the therapeutic relationships I have experienced. I'm not sure I would have developed the faith to trust in what God has to say about me, had it not been for therapy helping me get some unhealthy, competing beliefs out of His way.

Yes, I will always come to the end of me. Even the best therapies inevitably will have an end. But I will never come to the end of Jesus. And the freedom I want, the kind that lasts in this life *and* throughout eternity, can only be found in Him.

It is here that I will risk being redundant and say that if you have been leaning into your faith and looking for healing through spiritual means alone and are still struggling to break free from the grips of traumatic memories, emotional pain and relational dysfunction, then please seek the help of a gifted, clinically trained professional counselor. There is no shame in this. (And if you need medication to help as well, there is no shame in that either.) Consider this an act of faith in and of itself—trusting that therapy will work because it honors the way your brain is wired for processing, healing and change.

However, if you have tried therapy and/or medication, all the while excluding God from the equation, then it might be time to consider checking out the claims of Jesus and opening up to the idea of letting Him help you heal and break free.

YOUR TURN: Reflect. Engage. Write.

What, if any, has been your experience of how mental health is handled in Christian circles?

What, if any, has been your experience of how faith is handled in clinical/mental health settings?

Is faith an important part of your healing journey? If so, can you also see the value that therapy, in addition to faith, offers when working through complex issues of trauma and repeated patterns of dysfunction?

What, if anything, has held you back from seeking professional help?

What, if anything, has held you back from seeking out a relationship with Jesus as a part of your healing journey?

What are the benefits to addressing all aspects of our being when we are talking about healing? (Mental, emotional, physical and spiritual.)

Journal about a time when you personally experienced one facet influencing another, (i.e., when your spiritual affected your emotional or your physical influenced your mental, etc.)

Who can you share your thoughts with? If you are willing to take the next step into healing, will you consider asking them to be an encourager for you on the journey?

What is one step you are willing to take on your healing journey today?

PART EIGHT

A Word from Fellow Travelers

CHAPTER 21

Encouragement and Questions

Before we dive into Part Eight, let's check in. How are you doing?
No, ***really.*** How are you?

I wish we could be sitting together, eyeball to eyeball, so I could ask you in person how all that you've read so far is sitting with you. What a gift it would be to explore with you any "aha! moments" you may have about your own story as a result of reading mine.

Your responses to what came up in your own story might range from a sense of fondness over sweet memories to sorrow over the deepest of wounds. I wish we could be face to face so that I could tell you that I see you, I hear you and I believe you. And I am so sorry for the hurt you have endured.

Whatever your response, I do hope you grasp the importance of taking the journey through your own story like the one we have taken through mine. Perhaps you have already begun by following through on answering the questions in this book and journaling your responses. If so, keep going! And remember to be kind to yourself along the way.

Maybe you have read up to this point and are saying "this was a great exercise for you, Gina. But I don't really see much point to it for me."

And, if that *is* you, then, OK, I get it. But, if you will just humor me for a moment, I would like to share something with you.

First, I want to assure you my encouragement to understand your story is not some idea I have drummed up through my own process. You probably know as well as I do that there is now a myriad of studies we could cite which have shown a significant benefit to knowing and understanding our stories and, to some extent, the stories that contributed to them.

The work of Dr. Brené Brown, Dr. James Pennebaker, Dr. Dan Allender and Dr. Richard Schwartz, as well as a whole host of other mental health professionals, have presented significant research on the power of knowing (and telling) our story. And we can see in science, as well as in Scripture, the connection from generation to generation.

As Brené says, explore our pain… "not for the purpose of defining us. But for the purpose of being able to write a different ending." *If we so choose.*

It is not an overstatement to say that our story is one of the most significant things we possess. "Story" is one of the most profound means of communicating and understanding any of us have. Want to connect with someone regarding a similar experience? Tell a story. Want an effective way to teach a lesson? Tell a story. Want to share how you are feeling? You can do it effectively through story. Or, how about entertaining, offering hope, or motivation? Tell. A. Story. Jesus Himself taught through stories more than anything else.

And here is something else. It would seem there really *is* something to be said for writing down our stories—including our traumas. Dr. James Pennebaker's research shows us that writing about our lives, for as little

as 15 minutes in four sessions, improves our overall sense of health and well-being. Conversely, the research also shows that suppressing our stories and negative emotions impairs our overall health.

To add even more encouragement and inspiration, I wanted to share (with permission) some important contributions from others who have done this work of processing through their story and healing for themselves. The comments you are about to read are all from mental health professionals. They have not only taken this journey with many of their clients, but they have taken the journey personally for themselves. (As an aside, this makes them my favorite kind of therapists.)

I decided to share what they have to say on the subject because I believe it is helpful to hear the experiences of others. These Fellow Travelers have some important thoughts to share on what it was like to do the good, hard work of exploring past generations in their own families and I didn't want you to miss out on it.

Across the board, one question I consistently asked, without variation, was this: *"Was it worth it?"* And, the consistent answer? "Absolutely."

Now, let me be clear, your Fellow Travelers here discovered some difficult things about the generations that had gone before them. And many have yet to find full resolution to the questions they've asked.

Some said there were times during their process when they wished they had never begun the quest of discovery. But at the end of the day, they would not go back to not knowing. Across gender, age, racial and socioeconomic status, those I interviewed had some stunningly similar responses to my questions.

With their permission, I have included their initials but excluded their names for privacy. In the event they decide to read this one day, I wanted

them to know what they said mattered—perhaps more than they will ever know.

QUESTIONS AND ENCOURAGEMENTS FROM MY FELLOW TRAVELERS

"The question of 'how did I get here?' was answered for me when I began to uncover and understand past generations of my family. So much about the things I believed about myself that were unhelpful were a direct result of input from those who went before me." —M.P.

"I had faulted my parents for the chaos I endured as a kid. As I understood their stories, I began to forgive and understand the patterns of their behavior were consequences of what they went through as kids. They were truly doing the best they could do. I learned I could forgive them without denying the pain that I experienced in my childhood." —S.B.

"I wish someone would've said to me 'the pieces may not come together in your timing. Trust the process.' Often God protects us from knowing what we're not ready to know." —M.T.

"Understanding what my parents went through and some of what they passed on to me, even if they passed it implicitly, helps me understand why I get triggered by the things I do. And now, I have a plan for how to handle it." —K.J.

"I have come to a place of compassion, understanding and love. My inner work and the understanding of past generations brought me to that place. It feels freeing." —M.K.

"Doing work to uncover patterns in your family is important. It's what makes you who you are. You didn't get to be who you are from nothing." —I.M.

(This next comment will be the only quote I use from this fellow traveler who gave me permission to use his full name. I believe he deserves all the credit he's willing to accept for his contribution.)

Meet my friend, Michael Palanski.

"The truth is like water. It will find its way through."

Let me say it again...

> The truth is like water.
> It will find its way through.

You feel it too, right? It is one of those phrases that seeps down deep when you hear it, reverberating off the walls of your soul, demanding that its full weight be acknowledged.

Throughout the rest of our conversation, Michael peeled back the layers of his profound statement. He shared how he saw the past generations play out in the way he lived his own life. In the things he believed about himself and others. And I think he is on to something, because the same is true for me. It has been true for many I have worked with as well. Even without our explicit knowledge or awareness, they just sort of "show

up." But once we understand this, we then get to *decide* to learn just how they are showing up, and what we want to do about it.

One way will give us power. The other will take it away.

Which leads me to the last response I would like to share. It is my own and it came at the start of one my conversations when a colleague turned the tables in our interview. Before I could ask my first question, he asked one himself. "What called you to write a book about this subject?"

What called me...

Without realizing it, he had chosen the most accurate words possible to describe my inner state writing this book. Not driven or compelled. Drawn and propelled. Called.

As I worked through the difficult parts of my past, questions often arose about mom, dad, biological parents, stepparent, etc. And as I processed through traumas in my life, some of which I had never given myself permission to classify as traumas because I either thought they were my own fault or I didn't think they were severe enough to merit that label, I *learned* to believe that what happened to me was not because of something I did or did not do. My thinking about my life experiences really took a shift.

The only problem was that my acceptance of this new information was only at a head level. It had not penetrated the deeper parts of my heart and soul. There was always this little girl within me who wondered, "What if I was better, easier, quieter, louder, prettier, smarter, etc. Would things have been different?" She was too vulnerable and felt like a threat to my ability to heal, so I ignored her and pushed her aside. I did not want her insecurities and longings to get in the way of my success. I went full cognitive, rationalizing away her existence as being bothersome and

distracting. Ironically, that was the same thing that was done to me when I was an *actual* child.

It took me a long time to come to terms with the fact that I needed to love and embrace and integrate my inner child part as well as my rebellious adolescent part, and all those other "parts" that would act out or hide as a well-intentioned (albeit dysfunctional) means of protecting me. I needed all parts of myself to feel loved and valued. It was my only hope of becoming whole and wholly healed. BTW—In some ways, I believe that's a *perpetual* journey.

The unexpected bonus of this process was that I found a deeper sense of grace and compassion for the generations before me.

Giving myself permission to learn and understand the lives of generations before me, all the way back to my great grandparents, the things they endured as children and adolescents, allowed me to grieve it all differently. Healing moved from my head to my heart.

To be clear, this does not take away the fact that they were responsible for caring well for me and in many ways, they failed. But it does allow me to hold all of that in tension with grace, forgiveness, acceptance (which is *not* the same thing as agreement) and love.

Something I have come to realize is that one of our greatest gifts from God is one we abuse the most—our free will. While the generations before me were broken, it was their shattered pieces that cut *me* deeply. I recognize that the way they abused their free will to harm me was a result of their own pain and unresolved issues. It was not God's fault. He was neither culpable nor complicit. And I am confident that my pain grieved His heart.

And, so to answer my friend's question, *that* is what "called me" to write this book. When I get the privilege of using my story to bring

hope, encouragement or understanding to another? Well, *that* takes redemption this side of heaven to a new level. While pain shared is pain divided, healing shared is hope and freedom multiplied.

SHINING A LIGHT

Now, it's your turn. As you contemplate a deeper journey into your story and the story of those who have gone before you, here are some questions that might help you decide the course you wish to take. These are questions from colleagues and even a few from clients. Some are questions I asked myself as well. I will often use them to help clients consider whether or not they want to do the generational work in their own story.

As you consider these questions, I want you to consider something else. No matter how ready *you* are for this work in your story, it is possible that you will upset the *family system* when you begin to ask questions and connect dots. Do not let that surprise you. And please do not let it derail you either.

In all likelihood, your questions will shine light in places that remained dark for a very long time. In the same way that our eyes respond to light after spending time in the dark, the exposure can be painful, for you and for members of your family. Be ready for resistance and be ready to walk through it and to know when to move on. Who knows? In your quest for healing and understanding, you might set someone else free in the process.

Questions to Consider:

1. Can I be "OK" no matter what I uncover about my family or myself?

Of all the questions we can ask ourselves, this one will likely carry the most weight. It can be all too tempting to give a quick "yes" in response. But this question is too important to rush past. So please, go back and read it again. *Slowly.*

Now, let me explain what I mean by "OK."

In looking for information about your family, there is a chance you will discover things that are painful to hear. Some of it may be life changing. (I can say it was for me.) So, when I say, "can you be OK," I don't mean indifferent or numb. Almost unquestionably, you will be impacted by the information you hear.

What I mean is this: ***can you put systems and people in place for yourself to make sure that you're able to process through what you uncover and come out healthy on the other side?***

This might look like finding a counselor and processing through your own experiences (what you have already experienced or what you already know). It might look like confiding in your spouse, close friend(s) or someone else you trust who can check in with you along the journey. It might be someone who can pray with you, be your person when you find something out that you aren't sure what to do with, or when you find out something that feels like a missing piece to understanding yourself or others in your family.

Whatever it might need to look like for you, get these supports in place *before* you set out on your journey.

2. What is my motivation for uncovering the potential patterns in my family?

It is not up to me to tell you what those reasons *should* be. There isn't necessarily a right or wrong answer here (unless you want to know for the sake of gossip or harming someone, which would, of course, be wrong.) This is important. Knowing your "why" is important because it will help you stay motivated and committed.

3. How far back into the previous generations should I go?

For me, this was important because a lot of the patterns of behavior in my family started with my great grandparents. It was helpful to have

information on that generation. Science also seems to point to patterns of trauma and related responses impacting as far as the fourth generation, particularly without some sort of intervention. (Interestingly enough, the Bible seems to point to that same "third and fourth generation" impact.)

4. Who can/should I ask about my family?

The answer to this may not be as obvious as you think. It can be a struggle to sit face to face with family members, particularly when the relationship is strained or if it is unsafe for you to do so.

In my case, by the time I felt strong enough and ready to do this work, both my adopted and biological mothers had died. I had to piece together what I knew and then go on to friends and family members who had been there. Some of them I had not talked with since I was a child. Some I had not even remembered but connected with through Ancestry.com.

Then there were best friends of family members who had a front row seat to their formative years. Aunts, cousins, uncles—anyone can be a valuable resource if they were there and are willing. Just remember, it can be taboo to speak ill of the dead, so it might take some coaxing and explaining to get them to see the importance of any information they can offer. This of course becomes more complicated when you are asking about someone who is still alive. If you come upon a dead end, just remember—you do not have to know every part of the story to reveal deeper levels of understanding.

5. What present/past struggles have I experienced that I suspect have roots in previous generations of my family? (This can be part of your answer to "why do I want to do this work?")

Because I knew at least a few things about my family on my biological mother's side, I was able to see how patterns were repeating in my life that related to what occurred in previous generations. The more questions I asked, the more I was able to see how my beliefs, behaviors

and experiences were repeating from the generations before me. Like a photo mosaic, the smaller pictures, when viewed from a healthy distance, helped me see the bigger picture.

6. What did I experience in my childhood (what was I taught, how was I treated, what has contributed to the way I relate in my world, etc.), that may have been influenced by things that happened to my parents or my grandparents?

This goes back to what I said earlier in this chapter. It was difficult to come to terms with some of the developmental neglect, verbal and emotional abuse that I experienced as a child, and *not* wonder what it was about me that caused my parents and caregivers to act and react the way they did.

The realization of what my parents and grandparents endured (ALL of my parents), helped me see what contributed to their inability to parent me well. At the risk of over-emphasizing, I want to be clear (again) and say that still does not excuse away their behaviors. They still own the responsibility. But learning what I have allowed me to understand, to forgive and have grace and compassion towards them as wounded children who became wounded adults.

7. What will I do with this information?

I realize this may be a difficult question to answer. There is a likelihood you will not fully know what you *need* to do with it. But revisiting your "why" might be helpful.

For me, I wasn't interested in going on this journey for the sake of the journey itself. I wanted to know because I believed that the knowledge would help me heal and help me to know myself more. Knowing and understanding gave me a chance to help my kids see what obstacles might be in their way and to own my parenting mistakes and any pain I caused them so I might be able to do better, to *be* better for them.

I believed with everything in me that God was leading me along the way. So, when I came up against an impenetrable barrier to something I was trying to uncover, I would let it go. Because I also believe that in those moments, those pieces of information would have served only to distract or harm me or others.

And so it will be for you. In your journey, you will have to trust there may be times when God is shielding you from something or someone for one reason or another. Then move on to what you can discover and be ready for Him to help you see what you are supposed to do with the information.

8. Can I remember to look for good or fun traits/patterns/behaviors etc. that were passed down to me from generations gone by?

Learning the importance of this was sort of a happy accident for me. Turns out, it was the case for a few people I interviewed as well. Allowing yourself to see what you may have inherited that is fun or good or of value to you can soften the blows of what you discover that is more painful. Giving yourself permission to embrace the good things you find offers something redeeming in your inheritance.

For me it was discovering my love of writing, sense of justice, wanting to fight for those who cannot fight for themselves, helping others, resiliency and creativity were all pieces of my inheritance. All of which I am happy to say, have been passed on to my kids. Much of this I can see in my grandkids, too.

After meeting my father, I uncovered something a bit more daring that I inherited. When I was in my late teens, I owned a white Trans-Am and I *loved* to street race (*Don't Judge.*) As it turns out, I come from a long line of lead-footed, skillful female drivers, including my Aunt Sally who drove a white Trans-Am! Additionally, my biological father *literally* raced around the country when he was younger.

As you travel on your journey, it is my wish that you find some things within your inheritance that bring you joy as well.

I hope the questions in this section prove helpful as you plan your story work. Remember, it will be important to let your journey be just that: *yours.* Before you embark on the journey of asking questions in your family, please work through Part Nine of this book. The information will be invaluable in helping you build a framework for the questions you may want to ask and who you want to ask them of.

YOUR TURN: Reflect. Engage. Write.

Take some time to review the questions in this section and give yourself as much time as you need to answer them as best you can.

When you have finished, share what comes to mind with someone you trust. And if you are more of a verbal processor, consider inviting someone into the journey as you ponder the questions in this section.

Additionally, consider and journal on the following questions...

What is one thing you like about yourself that you inherited from a family member?

What is your biggest question for your family that you believe would have the greatest impact on you if you knew the answer?

Journal any additional thoughts or questions that came up for you while reading this portion of the book.

PART NINE
Your Turn

CHAPTER 22

Exploring and Expanding Your Journey

OK, My Brave Friend—now that you have heard examples from Fellow Travelers experienced in doing this deep generational work, and carefully considered some questions for the journey ahead, it is your turn to recognize the power of generational patterns, and the influence previous generations can have on how we see ourselves, others, the world around us and even God in your own life.

And if that is true, then I think you will find this section of great value. As we move forward through these next pages, I am going to ask you to trust me when I ask you to take the material in the order it is presented. I am not normally a stickler about these things, especially given the various sections and subject matter we are covering. But right here, in *this* portion, I ask that you kindly grant my request and proceed with the material in the order it's presented.

Before we dig in, I need to make sure you hear me loud and clear on something. No matter what you've been told or what you've read, including here in these pages, no one gets to tell you what has or hasn't had a life-changing, perspective-altering impact on your life except you.

You do not have to justify any of those circumstances to convince others of their validity. They do not have to be "bigger" than what other people have experienced, and they do not need to be quantifiable on any kind of scale other than their impact on your life.

It's important to call this out, because in my own experience and with many people I have worked with over the years, impactful events went unaddressed because somewhere along the way we came to believe they weren't big enough to be acknowledged for the painful events they were. Instead, it just heaped shame on top of the pain because we didn't believe it was acceptable to call those events what they were.

Traumatic.

It's also important to mention that while I want to help you give voice to significant events in your life and the lives of your family members, I don't want to help you build armor or walls around your story that you use to keep people out. I don't want you to use what you learn to justify staying in your own patterns of unhealthy beliefs and behaviors.

Acknowledge what has happened and the consequences of it, but do not stop there. Take the next brave step and find help to recover from it. Seek out the weapons you need to slay the shame and break the cycles in your own life so you can truly find freedom. My prayer is that in the process, you discover all kinds of possibilities to fully embrace who you have been created to be. Let the next portion of this book be one of the tools you use to get there.

EXPANDING YOUR PERSPECTIVE

To help you take a deeper look at events in your life and the lives of the generations before you, I thought it might be helpful to provide you with a lens to look through. Our lens comes in the form of two questionnaires

to help you think differently about traumas and events that could pose risk or harm to us as children.

Some of these questions may stir your memories or cause you to reflect on circumstances in your history in a way you have not previously considered. Although they are questions, this is *not* a test. When you feel that you are pressuring yourself to hurry up and move on to the next question, or when you feel overwhelmed by memories the question brings up: **STOP**.

When you find yourself seeing something in a new light, grab paper and pen and write what your heart needs to say. It does not matter if it makes much sense in the moment. It does not matter if it comes out in complete sentences. Just let it out. And if you feel yourself getting overwhelmed, set all of it aside and go do something that feeds your soul—preferably with *someone* who feeds your soul.

If you find you cannot get through these questions without deep, anxiety-producing pain, then please see that as a reason to seek out a trusted professional who can help you work through it all.

Questionnaire One

(Please note: Regarding the two questionnaires in this section, in the event that any of the questions asked stir memories or leave you feeling triggered in any way, remember to take special care of yourself. You can always put the book down, take a break, and come back when you are ready.)

Our first questionnaire is called **The A.C.E: The Adverse Childhood Experiences Questionnaire** (originally developed by Dr. Vincent Felitti). As you will see, the ACE Questionnaire addresses some of the more obvious things people consider when forms of childhood trauma are discussed.

As you engage with the ACE you will want a piece of paper so you can record your "score" (but remember this is *not* a test). Rather than writing in the book, you may want to record your yes and no answers in a separate location. But don't put too much stock in the actual *number*. This is more of a learning exercise.

Please remember that we are using this as a *guide*. I cannot stress strongly enough that these questions are not for the purposes of saying what does and doesn't count as a valid adverse experience.

It may also be worth noting that those who created the ACE and presented tremendous research over the years since its creation, did not intend for the inventory to be used as a definitive tool for validating categories of childhood trauma.

Finally, here are some additional pieces of information worth noting. According to the CDC's research using the ACE, two-thirds of American households have at least one of the topics mentioned in the ACE present. Further, one in five have three or more present. In practical terms, that means in a room of 100 people, 66 people have at least one of the categories in the ACE present, and 20 of those 100 present have three or more ACE categories present in their home.

It is important to note that according to research, having these situations as part of your early life experiences has been connected to a variety of issues in adolescents and adulthood like mental health issues, addiction and physical diseases. Some studies show there are over 40 medical conditions that are related to a person's adverse childhood experiences.

While these numbers may seem staggering, it is my hope that realizing the unfortunate prevalence of the experiences helps to destigmatize them, freeing you to be honest with your own answers in the inventory.

Adverse Childhood Experience (ACE) Questionnaire

While you were growing up, during your **first 18 years** of life:

1. Did a parent or other adult in the household often ... Swear at you, insult you, put you down, or humiliate you? (Or) Act in a way that made you afraid that you might be physically hurt?

   Yes **No** **If yes, enter 1 ______**

2. Did a parent or other adult in the household often ... Push, grab, slap, or throw something at you? (Or) Ever hit you so hard that you had marks or were injured?

   Yes **No** **If yes, enter 1 ______**

3. Did an adult or person at least 5 years older than you ever... Touch or fondle you or have you touch their body in a sexual way? (Or) Try to or actually have oral, anal, or vaginal sex with you?

   Yes **No** **If yes, enter 1 ______**

4. Did you often feel that ... No one in your family loved you or thought you were important or special? (Or) Your family did not look out for each other, feel close to each other or support each other?

   Yes **No** **If yes, enter 1 ______**

5. Did you often feel that ... You did not have enough to eat, had to wear dirty clothes and had no one to protect you? (Or) Your parents were too drunk or high to take care of you or take you to the doctor if you needed it?

   Yes **No** **If yes, enter 1 ______**

6. Were your parents ever separated or divorced?
   Yes **No** **If yes, enter 1 ______**

7. Was your mother or stepmother... Often pushed, grabbed, slapped or had something thrown at her? (Or) Sometimes or often kicked, bitten, hit with a fist or hit with something hard? (Or) Ever repeatedly hit over at least a few minutes or threatened with a gun or knife?

   Yes **No** **If yes, enter 1 ______**

8. Did you live with anyone who was a problem drinker or alcoholic or who used street drugs?

   Yes No If yes, enter 1 ______

9. Was a household member depressed or mentally ill or did a household member attempt suicide?

   Yes No If yes, enter 1 ______

10. Did a household member go to prison?

   Yes No If yes, enter 1 ______

Now add up your "Yes" answers: __________

This is your ACE "Score"

EXPANDING YOUR PERSPECTIVE (A LITTLE MORE)

I hope you were able to take that assessment without too much discomfort and I hope you remembered to care well for yourself in the process.

If you are feeling ready, let's dive right into our second guide.

This one is significant to us for a few reasons. While the ACE is helpful in some ways, many mental health professionals (myself included) recognize the list of questions on the ACE is not an exhaustive list when it comes to the events that we could consider as traumatic.

There is a strong body of research that children exposed to toxic stress and long-term stressors, brought about by "Big T" traumas (like categories on the ACE) and "Little t" traumas (like those that might seem less obvious), as well as exposure to unpredictable caregivers and unstable

home environments, can cause damage to the development and function of the brain.

Because the brain is exposed to high and/or constant levels of stress hormones in situations like these, learning and memory can be impaired, along with the ability to trust and have healthy relationships as adults. It can also impair a child's ability to trust even those who are trustworthy. In terms of memory and ability to trust, this was a dominant theme in my experience.

During adolescence and young adulthood, kids exposed to such traumas often turn to available substances for answers in lieu of getting professional help. Substances like nicotine, alcohol, marijuana and other drugs are used as a means of escaping how they're feeling; to relieve stress, anxiety, depression and even to deal with misplaced guilt and shame that might be associated with what happened to them as a child. Even things like high-risk sports, promiscuity and work/over-achievement, in childhood and adult life as well, might become a "drug of choice" to provide distraction from internal turmoil.

Any or all these behaviors, once developed as a means of coping, follow us into adulthood, causing all sorts of chaos and destruction when we want to be healthy and have healthy relationships. If this was a generational occurrence, it can be even more of a challenge to recognize what "healthy" really looks like.

At the end of the day, it's important to understand, and have validated, that a whole host of adverse childhood experiences have significant impact on our health: emotionally, mentally, physically and even spiritually, yes—in childhood and adolescence, but into adulthood as well.

Further, studies indicate health problems we experience as adults, related to these adverse circumstances in childhood and early life, are

most often treated merely at the symptoms-level, while the underlying cause (trauma) goes unaddressed. The root is not so readily recognized.

Some studies even show correlations, if not direct connections, to issues like auto-immune diseases, migraines, metabolic issues, intestinal distress of many forms, depression and/or anxiety and addictions with unaddressed consequences of trauma.

But the good news is, no matter what we have endured, the fact remains that our brains (and our lives) are very plastic. With the right interventions and relationships along with other resiliency factors, intrinsic or adapted, healing, growth and change are possible. And with them, freedom.

Which brings us to our second questionnaire.

Questionnaire Two

Because of the broad brush with which we can paint what classifies as a traumatic experience, I searched far and wide, having many conversations with a variety of mental health professionals in search of something that I could use to help you get your arms around it. But to no avail.

So, since I could not *find* what I was looking for, I decided to create it, with the help of others in my field. To make it happen, I enlisted the help of my trusted friend and colleague, David Koch, LPC. David is a therapist at CrossRoads Counseling Centers in St. Louis, Missouri. He formerly worked in a hospital setting running both individual and group therapy for those recovering from addictions, many of his clients having had some of the traumas identified in our questionnaire.

He is also an adjunct professor at Covenant Theological Seminary in their Counseling Program, teaching their Addictions Course. While he specializes in recovery, he also works with young adults, people

struggling through anxiety, depression, and mood concerns, and with men experiencing sexual brokenness.

David also works with spouses and parents who are wrestling through the struggles presented from the addiction or mental illness of a family member. He recognizes firsthand the importance of generational influences and the need to break those unhealthy cycles.

Together, David and I had the privilege of locking arms with approximately ***60*** other mental health professionals, to create **The Expanded Trauma Perspective Questionnaire** for the specific purpose of this book. You should know that their contributions came not only as the result of the work they have done with clients, but the work they have done in their own stories as well. We are so grateful for the participation of each and every one of them.

It is also our greatest hope that individuals and other mental health professionals will see **The Expanded Trauma Perspective Questionnaire** as a tool to help their clients discover some possible influencers that might otherwise go unrecognized for the impact they have had.

As David puts it,

> *"In the process of my counseling and teaching career, I've found that many people just don't recognize the trauma in their stories because much of it 'falls through the cracks.' This seems to be in part because they (and people around them) would not 'count it' as traumatic because it doesn't fall into what we might call traditional categories of trauma in its severest forms.*
>
> *I have watched people struggle with feeling conflicted and even guilty as they start to identify their experiences as 'traumatic,' which is why I wanted to join you to create this questionnaire.*

> *The process called to mind my own personal experience of that same kind of minimization and confliction in working through my own story that we are attempting to address with our work here. Specifically, when I was reading about trauma in counseling and started naming some of my family of origin experiences as traumatic and wounding, I remember a friend commenting that I needed to 'get over it' stating, 'it's not like your parents beat you.'*
>
> *I remember thinking that I wished there were physical markers to the pain I felt because I started to feel crazy that I felt so injured by events that left no noticeable wounds. But, in reality, they're more noticeable than we realize, if we know how to look for the scars."*

So, to you, my Dear, Brave Friend, From David, our trusted colleagues who participated in this endeavor, and myself, thank you for being the motivation and reason we did this work. We hope it will help you and many others beyond this book to look at trauma in a whole new light.

The Expanded Trauma Perspective Questionnaire

Place a check next to as many items as apply to your experience in each category, even if you checked a previous description that partially accounted for your experiences.

WIDELY RECOGNIZED EXPERIENCES OF TRAUMA

____ I experienced physical violence from a parent or sibling.

____ I experienced sexual attention (implicit or explicit) or contact from a family member.

____ I experienced uninvited sexual attention (implicit or explicit) or contact from another person.

____ There was physical violence against one of my parents/caregivers by the other.

____ My parents separated/divorced.

____ There was verbal, emotional or mental abuse in my home (parent to parent/parent to you/parent to sibling/sibling to sibling).

____ Someone in my home dealt with mental illness or attempted suicide.

____ Someone in my home was incarcerated.

UNDER-RECOGNIZED SOURCES OF TRAUMA

One or both of my parents/caregivers had a drug and/or alcohol problem (diagnosed or suspected) that caused any of the following in my home:

____ Unsteady work or loss of job.

____ Fighting between parents.

____ Emotional instability or lack of safety.

____ Physical or sexual abuse toward anyone in the family.

____ Verbal abuse.

____ Screaming or rage.

____ Destructive behavior like punching walls or breaking things.

One or both of my parents/caregivers had a mental illness (diagnosed or suspected) that caused any of the following in my home:

____ Unsteady work or loss of job.

____ Fighting between parents.

____ Emotional instability or lack of safety.

____ Physical or sexual abuse toward anyone in the family.

____ Verbal abuse.

____ Screaming or rage.

____ Destructive behavior like punching walls or breaking things.

THESE DESCRIBE MY EXPERIENCE(S) AS A CHILD: (Any item that ends with (+) is considered a contributor to resilience.)

____ It was OK to cry growing up. (+)

____ I felt comforted when I was upset. (+)

____ It was OK to make mistakes as a child. (+)

____ I felt safe to respectfully disagree. (+)

____ I got what I needed physically (food/clothing/shelter/clean and safe home/bed to sleep in) on a consistent basis. (+)

____ I received an adequate level of emotional nurturing from my mother. (+)

____ I received an adequate level of emotional nurturing from my father. (+)

____ Someone close to me (care giver, parent, sibling, etc.) dealt with an addiction.

____ My mother/father was emotionally unpredictable.

____ Another caregiver in the home was emotionally unpredictable.

____ I feared physical violence but never received it.

____ I tried to anticipate my parents/caregiver's mood and adapted my behaviors accordingly.

____ There was physical violence against a sibling(s) in my home.

____ My sibling(s) often hit me, touched me inappropriately or bullied me.

____ My parent(s) remarried or lived with a new significant other.

____ A significant person in my life questioned/changed sexual orientation or gender identity.

____ I was treated as a parent for my sibling(s) by my parent(s).

____ My family dealt with poverty.

____ There was at least one change in the person who had primary custody of me.

____ I had to move frequently; my living situation was unstable.

____ One or both of my parents had multiple romantic/relationship partners.

IN ONE OR MORE SIGNIFICANT RELATIONSHIPS (caregiver, family member, teacher, partner) **I HAVE OFTEN HEARD STATEMENTS LIKE:**

____ "What is wrong with you?"

____ "You're stupid!"

____ "Just shut up!"

____ "I'll smack/slap/punch you!"

____ "I'll give you something to cry about!"

____ "Stop crying!"

____ "Why aren't you more like your (sibling/friend)?"

____ "You're weird!"

____ "You don't fit in."

____ "You're too much . . ."

____ "You're not enough . . ."

____ "You're too sensitive!"

____ "You're just like your dad/mom!"

HOW WAS ANGER HANDLED IN MY HOME?

____ My parent(s) was silent/cut off communication when angry.

____ My parent(s) withheld love/affection when angry.

____ My parent(s) screamed regularly when angry.

____ Parent(s)/Sibling(s) threw things/slammed doors when angry.

____ Parent(s)/Sibling(s) took out anger on an innocent bystander (cursed/threatened/etc.).

____ Parent(s)/Sibling(s) took out anger physically on another or me (grabbed at, pulled hair, slapped/punched, etc.).

____ My caregiver made excuses for/minimized another caregiver's anger.

____ Arguments were discussed and/or repairs were made in relationship after negative behaviors. (+)

____ My parents apologized for their anger (anger was not inappropriate). (+)

WHAT DID DISCIPLINE LOOK LIKE GROWING UP?

____ I was hit by parent(s)/sibling(s) with an object in anger.

____ I was hit with a hand in anger.

____ Punishments were excessive.

____ Punishments were appropriate. (+)

____ I was verbally berated (by parent/teacher/coach/sibling) for mistakes.

____ I was rationally talked to about my misbehavior. (+)

____ I was taught what went wrong and how to make it right. (+)

____ Parent(s) would spank, one time, and in a calm manner (before the age of 10). (+)

DID I HAVE HEALTH CONCERNS AS A CHILD?

____ Surgery before age two.

____ Significant illness before age two.

____ Illness that caused extended hospital stay(s) or separation from mother/caregiver.

____ Surgery, illness or medical condition that went under or over treated.

____ Medical procedures (including surgery) without proper anesthesia.

____ Traumatic medical experience(s) with doctor, hospital, caregiver, etc.

FAITH/BELIEF IN GOD WHILE GROWING UP:

____ I was raised to be fearful/afraid of God.

____ God was presented as vengeful or all-punishing.

____ I was taught God is loving and forgiving. (+)

____ There was no spirituality in my childhood home.

____ We were part of a healthy church family growing up. (+)

____ I saw godly behaviors modeled by parent(s). (+)

____ I was told "You're not good enough for God."

____ I was taught you have to work hard to be good enough for God.

____ I was taught that God only chooses/loves good people.

____ I was raised to believe God is unapproachable.

____ My past/mistakes are too extreme for God to love me.

____ I was told to not bother God with little problems.

____ God was not there for me growing up.

____ I was taught about an impersonal God.

____ My parents did not agree on the concept of God.

Total number of items checked (excluding the (+) items) ________

Total number of items checked with (+) ________

Now that you have your numbers calculated, you are probably wondering what it means. Remember, the goal in participating in this questionnaire is to broaden your perspective of what might classify as "trauma" in your life or the life of another. There is not a standard to compare it to.

The goal in working through this questionnaire is to expand your ideas about what might have previously been unrecognized as trauma(s) in your life. It is my hope that you will feel validated as well as encouraged to take

the next step, which would be to find a professional to help you process through what you have learned in answering these questionnaires.

But…

Even if you didn't check a single thing on either of these questionnaires, and you have memories of things that you saw, or things said or done which caused a wounding in your heart and soul, or fed into an unhealthy belief about who you are, or caused you to doubt your great worth, or has contributed in some way to unhealthy patterns of relating to others, then that is valid and I want to see you get the support you need to heal.

On the flip side, you might look at the amount of statements that are true for you and feel hopeless or defeated. You might experience your higher number to be a signal that you are beyond help. (P.S. If you are breathing, you are capable of healing.) In either case, what I hope I am making abundantly clear is that the *number doesn't matter.*

"Then why give us the inventory in the first place?"

I am so glad you asked! Because I want you to be thinking on a global scale, not only about what might have impacted *your* life, but what may have impacted those who went *before* you.

In a pull-yourself-up-by-your-bootstraps-and-just-get-over-it society, it can be all too easy to gloss over or even bury experiences from your past, preventing you from seeing their influence in the life you're living today. The idea of the questionnaires is to help you think more concretely about this, for yourself and for your family of origin. Questions like these can also serve as guides to help you decide what sort of questions you might want answers to about generations before you. Questions like the ones included here are often related to the areas where secrets are kept in a family.

YOUR TURN: Reflect. Engage. Write.

What was the experience of taking the questionnaires like for you?

Were there any revelations that occurred to you as the result of participating in the questionnaires, and if so, what were they?

How has taking these questionnaires changed your ideas about what would be considered a traumatic experience?

Are you feeling a greater level of validation after taking these questionnaires?

How are you feeling after working through this portion of the book?

What will you do to take good care of yourself after engaging with these questionnaires?

Who is someone you can share your experience with?

THEIR TURN

Now that you have had a chance to take a deeper look into your own experiences, I'd like you to try something that has proved helpful for me and for many of my clients. On the same sheet of paper where you wrote your responses to our questions, I would like you to make six additional columns, assigning a column for each of the following: "Mom, Dad, Grandma/Grandpa (Paternal); Grandma/Grandpa (Maternal)." Do the same for great-grandparents as well but only if you know anything about them, or if you have access to someone who does. (The same holds true for all the names listed. Only include people you have some knowledge of, or those whom you can learn about from another source.)

Armed with whatever knowledge you presently have about these past generations, go back and take the **ACE** and **The Expanded Trauma Perspective Questionnaire** for each of the names listed on your paper.

I know that might seem like a strange request, but remember in Part Seven where I shared the responses from other mental health professionals who had done their own family of origin work and how powerful the experience were for them? Well, I want to give you an opportunity to have that same kind of experience using the tools I'm providing. It is my hope that answering these questions for your parents, and your parents' parents, and so on, will help you with that.

In my own personal experience, I can tell you that it was a healing exercise for me (although it was a bit clumsier for me as I didn't have questionnaires to help guide me.) Slowing down to really look at some of the things that those who have gone before me experienced not only helped me see where some of those unhealthy, automatic thoughts and reactions in life came from (I *learned* them. Which meant I could *unlearn* them.), but it also helped me see what each of them was working with that informed what they contributed to my life.

If you think about it, everything we believe about ourselves, relationships, spirituality, health, diet, politics, social issues, how we treat our fellow man (or woman), literally e-v-e-r-y-t-h-i-n-g begins in *our* "beginning" and is informed by those who are closest to us and responsible for helping us learn and grow. Learning about those who were most influential in our lives helps us determine what we may want to challenge as being true, or completely dismantle to rebuild a healthier perspective.

In my experience, seeing how my family's brokenness perpetuated brokenness was powerful. It helped me understand, at a deeper level,that the negative impact of their behaviors on my life were completely on them and those before them, not the result of something I did or failed to do as a child.

It also helped me come to terms with that fact that God's heart grieved for the way others abused their free will to abuse and neglect me. God was neither complicit nor culpable. It was broken people suffering the consequences of broken people abusing their free will, generation to generation. It was also about them failing to make the changes necessary to stop the cycle—which sort of makes sense. You can't heal what you can't see.

But none of what I have learned lets anyone off the hook in terms of excusing their bad behavior. It didn't minimize how it impacted me. Nor did it invalidate what happened to me. I was still wounded. I still had a lot of recovery to do.

Yet, what I learned allowed me to create a *new* cycle, one of compassion and healing. As I found compassion for each of them, I found more space for more healing. Then more compassion, for them and for myself. Then, more healing.

YOUR TURN: Reflect. Engage. Write.

What was the experience like for you in taking these questionnaires on behalf of the generations before you?

Were there any shifts in how you feel about any particular member(s) of your family? If so, take a moment to write down how you felt about them before, and how you're feeling now.

Did any repeated patterns reveal themselves in this process? If so, what were they?

What were some "Aha" moments you experienced as you participated in this exercise?

PAIN OUTSIDE THE FAMILY

While there were several abusive experiences in my life perpetrated by people *not* in my family, I do believe my healing journey would have been much different had there been a stable and supportive family around whom I trusted to tell what had happened. But that's part of the point I am trying to make here. They were unable to be what *I* needed them to be because *they* were not given what *they* needed. It doesn't make it right. But it is the truth of how it was.

Giving grace and releasing the hurt might be hard for you to think about. Maybe you are not there yet. Maybe my perspective on the whole thing is unsettling for you. If that is the case, I get it. This is another place where I wish we could sit, eyeball to eyeball and talk about it.

But, since we might not ever get the chance, I want to make sure to let you know that I hear you, and I see you and I am sorry you were harmed. More than anything else, I *really* want to see you set free from any further harm.

RESILIENCY CAN BE GENERATIONAL TOO

As much as it's important to understand the circumstances that might've contributed to our lives in a negative way, it is equally important (and some would argue even *more important)* to understand what has contributed to our lives in a positive way. Those *are* the things we want to hang on to. Those are the traits we *want* to pass on from generation to generation. And those are key factors in determining our resilience, healing and growth.

We have already explored one aspect that builds resiliency: Emotionally Corrective Experiences. Hopefully, you were able to identify a few of those from your own life. (If you didn't engage in an exercise to identify

any of those experiences in your life when you read through that section the first time, please take some time to do so now. It's OK. I will wait.)

Now I would like us to look at a guide for helping assess what has contributed to our resilience. (Oh! And—My Strong Friend, just in case you do not think of yourself as resilient, the fact that you chose to read this book proves that you are.) Predictably, the tool we will use to explore this idea is called **The Resilience Questionnaire**.

The Resilience Questionnaire was created in 2006 with revisions in 2013. The lead authors of the questionnaire are psychologists Mark Rains and Kate McClinn. It was modeled after the ACE and the content was created based on numerous studies (although the questionnaire itself is not intended for research purposes). According to Rains, the main goal of the RQ is to *"prompt reflection on topics that may be protective and improve a person's resiliency."*

Since this questionnaire was written with the intention of serving as a prompt for deeper reflection, please take your time going through the statements. It may even help to read them twice. Make sure to record your answers on a separate sheet of paper or in your journal.

As with our previous questionnaires, please remember the RQ is meant to serve as a guide to help us recognize what kind of things contribute(d) to our resilience. I chose this guide because first, it can help us see the positives we hadn't given full weight to in the past. Secondly, it can point us to what we should seek to provide for our children or even grandchildren, no matter what age they are. In the here and now, we can even provide some of these things for ourselves as well.

As you read through **The Resilience Questionnaire** it is likely you will have memories of people and situations that fit the theme of the statements. Please take the time to write down those experiences! I cannot stress this enough. In all likelihood, you will find some of these

memories can lead you to your Emotionally Corrective Experiences. At a minimum, they reinforce the positive self-narrative that is so essential to embracing the redemptive truth about ourselves.

For example, were I exploring statements seven and twelve for the first time (see RQ below), they would each give me the opportunity to reflect on the influence of Sister Debbie in my life, which would lead me to explore an important ECE in my life as well.

This may also be a questionnaire to revisit from time to time, particularly if you are working with a counselor to process your story. It may be that you will see and understand things differently once you have had an opportunity to process and heal.

The Resilience Questionnaire

Please circle the most accurate answer under each statement:

1. **I believe that my mother loved me when I was little.**

   Definitely True   Probably True   Not Sure   Probably Not True   Definitely Not True

2. **I believe that my father loved me when I was little.**

   Definitely True   Probably True   Not Sure   Probably Not True   Definitely Not True

3. **When I was little, other people helped my mother and father take care of me and they seemed to love me.**

   Definitely True   Probably True   Not Sure   Probably Not True   Definitely Not True

4. **I have heard that when I was an infant someone in my family enjoyed playing with me, and I enjoyed it too.**

   Definitely True   Probably True   Not Sure   Probably Not True   Definitely Not True

5. **When I was a child, there were relatives in my family who made me feel better if I was sad or worried.**

   Definitely True   Probably True   Not Sure   Probably Not True   Definitely Not True

6. **When I was a child, neighbors or my friends' parents seemed to like me.**

   Definitely True   Probably True   Not Sure   Probably Not True   Definitely Not True

7. **When I was a child, teachers, coaches, youth leaders or ministers were there to help me.**

   Definitely True   Probably True   Not Sure   Probably Not True   Definitely Not True

8. **Someone in my family cared about how I was doing in school.**

   Definitely True   Probably True   Not Sure   Probably Not True   Definitely Not True

9. **My family, neighbors and friends talked often about making our lives better.**

   Definitely True   Probably True   Not Sure   Probably Not True   Definitely Not True

10. **We had rules in our house and were expected to keep them.**

    Definitely True   Probably True   Not Sure   Probably Not True   Definitely Not True

11. **When I felt really bad, I could almost always find someone I trusted to talk to.**

Definitely True Probably True Not Sure Probably Not True Definitely Not True

12. **As a youth, people noticed that I was capable and could get things done.**

Definitely True Probably True Not Sure Probably Not True Definitely Not True

13. **I was independent and a go-getter.**

Definitely True Probably True Not Sure Probably Not True Definitely Not True

14. **I believed that life is what you make it.**

Definitely True Probably True Not Sure Probably Not True Definitely Not True

15. **As a child and/or youth, there was an adult present to support me in times of struggle.**

Definitely True Probably True Not Sure Probably Not True Definitely Not True

How many of the 15 protective factors above did you circle "Definitely True" or "Probably True"? _____

Of these circled, how many are still true for you? _____

If you were able to find even one of these statements that are true for you, then you are resilient! It is possible, and even probable, that more of these answers can become true over time. Our perspectives shift with understanding and healing.

If you struggled with this questionnaire, please try not to feel defeated. I too struggled the first time I was asked questions similar to these. I was so broken that I would have only been able to agree with *one* of these statements. And agree half-heartedly at that. But as my perspective shifted and I worked through the more difficult portions of my story, I

was able to see things differently. It is my hope you will be able to do that too.

You can also consider some of the ways in which you can build resiliency now—things like working on acceptance and optimism, discovering and enhancing your strengths, building relationships with people who lift you up and develop a sense of curiosity and humor. Any and all of these can help rewire our brains and build our resilience. And, as always, the journey is best taken with a trusted friend and perhaps a professional counselor.

One more thing before we move on. I want to share that one of the most helpful relationships that had helped me build my resiliency has been my relationship with Jesus.

Looking back, I can see that the portions of my journey which I attempted to take without Him were much darker and produced less healing and growth than those portions with Him.

YOUR TURN: Reflect. Engage. Write.

In what ways has taking **The Resilience Questionnaire** helped you recognize the power you have to overcome challenges?

What are some ways you can intentionally build resiliency in your own life and help your kids/grandkids/etc. build resiliency as well?

List some of the specific things in your life that have contributed to resiliency, things that might not even be on the questionnaire.

What resiliency traits have you seen in your family members?

Can you see any heredity in those traits? If so, where and how?

PART TEN

Therapy Things

CHAPTER 23

Thoughts on (Some) Therapies that Help

(You didn't think we'd get through this book without exploring this—at least a little bit—did you?)

> For some people, the word "therapy" alone engenders a butt-scrunch moment.

You may literally have a visceral reaction to this topic. And if so, I get it. The idea of opening up to a stranger and daring to let light shine on our most difficult moments can feel overwhelming. While there is an abundance of qualified professionals out there, sadly, therapy can get a bad name.

As we discussed in the Part Seven (*Jesus and a Therapist*), those of us who are followers of Jesus have likely been exposed to some frustrating perspectives in the Christian community regarding mental health. In the quest for healing, many have been told (or made to feel) that the *real* problem is a lack of faith or a sin problem.

Having said all of that, I don't want you to use those negative experiences as a reason to push God out of your healing journey or give up on getting help. You can *absolutely* find a clinically trained therapist with a redemptive worldview, rooted in Christ, who will work with you on your healing. I promise you *they* ***are*** *out there*! I know because I had a few of them help me in my life. I get to call many of them "colleague and friend." As you may recall, several of them were part of the group who helped us create the questionnaire in the previous section. (Oh, and also, I *am* one of those therapists.)

As for the types of therapy that you might find helpful, there are many out there that take wonderful and creative approaches. Good counseling, in part, helps us adjust our lenses so we can learn to see relationships from a healthier perspective. Some therapies can even teach us, in practical, life-applicable ways, the skills we need to be emotionally regulated and effective in our relationships with others, ourselves and even God.

But always (a word that I do not use lightly), counseling/therapy, whatever you want to call it, should feel like something you are doing *with* your therapist. If it feels more like something is being done *to* you, have a conversation with your counselor. And if it does not change, you may need to find a new one. You want a partner for the journey, not someone who merely draws you a map and tells you where to go.

THOUGHTS ON THERAPEUTIC APPROACHES

While so much of life's struggles are *felt* on a heart level, much of the battle we face from day to day is in our mind. Not that we have made up or imagined our experiences, pain, and struggles. What I mean is that because our experiences can impact the way we relate to everything and everyone, our mind is typically the battlefield where we attempt to make sense of our emotions, then respond or react accordingly.

It can be overwhelming to sort out what "healthy" looks like amidst the many unhealthy experiences earlier in life. Changing our perspectives and beliefs, learning to trust others and even God, (not to mention-learning to trust ourselves) can feel like an insurmountable task. But just because it *feels* that way, doesn't make it true. And this is where Science is catching up to what Scripture has told us all along. It is possible to create change. We can literally be transformed by the renewing of our minds (Romans 12:2). We can flip the script on our self-narrative. (*"As a person thinks in their hearts, so they shall be." Proverbs 23:7)* Change is not only possible, but often, that unsettled feeling we experience is the craving of our soul for change; for things to be different, to be whole and healed.

> Change is not only possible, but often, that unsettled feeling we experience is the craving of our soul for change . . .

While we don't have time or space here to cover the profound research available out there, you can check out the work of individuals like Dr. Richard Schwartz, Dr. Dan Siegel, Dr. Joe Dispenza, Dr. Caroline Leaf, Dr. Curt Thompson and the like for deeper conversations on all of the exciting findings of interpersonal neurobiology and our brains' ability to change.

But we do need to throw in a caveat, something that does not always get the attention it deserves. It's easy to get excited about the idea of changing our brains, because at first glance, this approach seems to say we have all the control over the thoughts we think and where they come from or how they impact us. What we are learning, however, is that this isn't always the case.

The reality is that in addition to working from a "top down" approach, where the battle is mostly fought in the mind, we need to be aware of and enlist help in exploring our need for incorporating a "bottom up" approach as well. By that, I mean sometimes, the work we need to do is

much deeper than what we can access on a cognitive level. It is visceral. We must pay attention to what is happening in our bodies as well as our minds. This was a critical piece in my own healing as well.

Many of us have had traumatic experiences that were harmful enough to cause our cognitive, rational, reason-making portions of our brains (think parts of the brain associated with thinking, speaking, and current emotional awareness) to shut down for the sake of protection. In those situations, the much older portions of the brain (those responsible for things like reflexes, memories, and automatic survival responses) took over to try and ensure our survival.

Sometimes those experiences are stored in the body, so enlisting therapies that approach healing from a strictly cognitive or talk-based approach fall short. There can also be traumas that occur preverbal, or perhaps trans-generationally, the likes of which we cannot make sense of because we simply have no context for it. In those cases, taking a talk-based or cognitive approach alone can be harmful.

Some of the authors I mentioned earlier take this bottom up approach into account. Additionally, authors like Dr. Bessel Van der Kolk, Dr. Gabor Mate, Dr. Peter Levine and Dr. Francine Shapiro have given us tremendous resources as therapists to help us think through the concept of including body sensations and that bottom up approach. If you're interested in the topic, I would suggest taking a look at some of their research and practice philosophies.

As we think about the combination of faith and therapy, we must remember that we are multifaceted beings: emotional, mental, physical and spiritual. The most successful therapies recognize that integration is key and the modalities of therapy that bring us the most success are those that take all parts of our being into account. Good therapy asks the question, *"What has happened to you and how were you able to survive it?"* And *great* therapy says, *"Let's find the best way to help you*

heal from your experiences and do so in a manner that honors the whole of who you are."

To round out the theme of what quality therapy looks and feels like, we know we are receiving it when we feel seen and affirmed, that our behavior makes sense in light of what happened to us, even if that behavior has become maladaptive and destructive.

This is incredibly freeing because it helps eliminate the shame that can come when we can't make reason out of the things we do and the ways we react. It frees us to say, *"Yes, that* ***does*** *make sense in light of what happened to me. But as I learn to recognize the relationships that I am truly safe in, I no longer want nor need to react in the ways I did when I didn't feel safe."*

THERAPEUTIC FAVORITES (SO FAR)

While I would love to speak expansively on all the solid therapies out there, in the interest of space, I will touch only on a few of my personal favorites. The therapies I included here are the ones I have found helpful for myself and/or with clients. These therapies have been recognized as some of the most effective approaches being used today. Of course, do not let that deter you from researching what else is out there. Take the time to find a counselor/therapist that fits with your personality and style of relating and allow that person to help you explore therapeutic options that are right for your needs.

Now, let's look at a few of my favorite therapies to help you think about what your own healing journey might look like.

Talk Therapy and Group Therapy

Talk Therapy and Group Therapy are more "umbrella" terms than anything else. The definition lies within that of psychotherapy, which is defined by the American Psychological Association (APA) as "the process in which therapists apply scientifically validated procedures to help people develop healthier, more effective habits." These therapies can be done in an individual setting, as well as in group. Sometimes you will hear the term "process group" in relation to group-talk therapy as well.

Talk Therapy allows the therapist and clients to collaborate on the healing journey. Much of what you read from here on will at least in part fall under this umbrella. Having a rapport with your therapist and feeling like you can "talk it out with them" is a critical piece to having success in therapy. It is worth noting that in some instances, "talk therapy" can be experienced with a trusted friend, pastor or mentor, as well as a mental health professional. While it may not be a substitute for counseling, do not discount the importance of having people in your life with whom you can be 100 percent your authentic self.

Both Group and Talk Therapies call to mind concepts in Scripture that refer to ideas like Ecclesiastes 4:9-10a "Two are better than one, because they have a good return for their labor: If either of them falls down, one can help the other up."

CBT

This therapy may be most familiar to you. Cognitive Behavioral Therapy (CBT) takes its direction from the interrelation of your social factors and individual thoughts and behaviors to help you improve your quality of life. It focuses on respectfully challenging unhelpful beliefs and behaviors to promote change. CBT can help you improve your emotional regulation (think responsive rather than reactive) and develop personal coping strategies to help you solve current problems.

In a nutshell, CBT works from the idea that our thoughts affect the way we feel and the way we feel affects the way we respond. The concept of CBT aligns well with ideas we see in Scriptures like our previously mentioned text, Romans 12:2, which instructs us to be "transformed by the renewing of our mind."

CBT was tremendously beneficial to me by helping me challenge much of what I assumed was true about myself and even about others. It helped me break down many unhealthy beliefs that had formed as the result of what I experienced and saw modeled in my family of origin (the family I grew up in.) I appreciated this approach because it offered practical therapy with skills and tools that I could utilize to live a more effective life.

Additionally, CBT offers ways to help manage stress and anxiety by learning relaxation techniques such as deep breathing and positive self-talk to help you cope, such as "I've done hard things before. I can do this." CBT also offers strategies to help you overcome avoidance, as well as communication skills for improving relationships.

Something to consider: CBT is not primarily focused on taking an in-depth look at your story. However, some exploration of story is helpful to make informed choices about what interventions will be most helpful for you. Regardless of what type of therapy you decide is right for you, many of them will have at least some small component of CBT included.

EMDR

EMDR is a therapy I wish I had known about sooner in my own personal journey. EMDR stands for Eye Movement Desensitization and Reprocessing. It has come a long way since its creator, Dr. Francine Shapiro, began the therapy in the late 1980's. It has expanded from eye movement (following a lightbar or finger moving from left to right) to also

using tapping, tones, or any combination of the former to help clients find healing.

In my experience, EMDR was a critical part of the healing journey. As much as CBT offered me a way to talk through and challenge some unhealthy perspectives, thoughts and beliefs, EMDR helped me work through the deeper pain I carried that was attached to the traumas and resulting shame.

In a nutshell, EMDR works to change maladaptive networks in the brain by connecting traumatic memories with new, helpful information. Distressing thoughts and emotions are sort of "disconnected" from the actual event they were created in, allowing a person to process through an event, or perhaps even a disconnected belief or emotion until there is no longer distress attached to the thought.

Lisa describes it like this: "When someone experiences a traumatic event, the distressing thoughts, emotions and other material associated with the event are sort of "disconnected" from normal healthy brain processing. EMDR therapy jumpstarts a person's brain processing system and allow the brain to work through the traumatic material (which could include a negative self belief. difficult emotions, or body sensations), until there is no longer distress attached to the event."

While there is the greatest body of research on EMDR as it pertains to PTSD, I would say just about anyone in need of processing unhealthy, unhelpful or harmful emotions or previous experiences would benefit from EMDR. *However,* the success of EMDR depends largely in part on the therapist and the perspective from which they have been trained, and the skillset they have developed.

To help us understand this better, I had the privilege of interviewing one of the top clinicians and trainers of EMDR. Lisa Sager, LPC. (Incidentally,

I was fortunate enough to sit under Lisa during my EMDR therapy training to become an EMDR practitioner.)

Lisa is a Missouri Licensed Professional Counselor and EMDR International Association Certified Therapist, Approved Consultant and EMDR Therapy Training Provider. With 20 years of EMDR therapy expertise, she has successfully treated a wide range of life adversities and trauma reactions, including Depression, Anxiety, PTSD, Complex/Developmental Trauma, Personality and Dissociative Disorders. Lisa also developed and directs the EMDR Training Center to provide creative and comprehensive trauma-informed education for mental health professionals internationally.

"It's a little awkward and difficult to explain the complexities of EMDR in a brief, graspable way," explains Lisa. "I would say the short version is that it helps to alleviate difficult emotions and body sensations that are stored in the body and brain, in ways other therapies can't."

When asked about the reasons clients seek EMDR Therapy, Lisa states, "It can be anything that causes disruptions in a person's healthy development, mentally and emotionally, and continues to cause problems throughout life." (I realize that sounds broad, but remember, we expanded on our definition of "trauma" during the assessment portion of this book. If you skipped it initially, now might be a good time to go back and engage with that material.)

"One of the things I really appreciate about EMDR is how it works on areas we can't really get to any other way," Lisa shares. "For example, pre-verbal trauma, or trauma that happens without the cognitive part of our brain online, is difficult to address with talk therapy. Trauma stored in emotional and physical centers of the brain needs more than conversation to be released."

A fascinating element of EMDR is that it can allow a person to process through something that once had deep emotional roots attached, so that it becomes a "mere thought." "EMDR also works on more than just specific events. We can see its efficacy for generational issues, and beliefs or thoughts we hold about ourselves, that may not seem clearly connected to any particular event in our lives."

This means what we carry from previous generational influences can also be released through therapies like EMDR. The result is that we can effectively break those cycles.

For some people, their entire lives were like a melting pot of chaos, with multiple traumas, big and small combined. "Sometimes, the traumas are about things that *didn't* happen as much as they are about the things that did," adds Lisa. "It can be completely body-based, meaning there is no actual event attached to what a person is experiencing emotionally."

According to Lisa, research shows, "You don't need to know or understand a person's whole story for EMDR to be effective. It is great for dealing with clients who have gaps in their history or holes in their memories. You can simply deal with whatever it is they bring. Sometimes it's spoken, sometimes there are no words. *This therapy can work with very little said.* In fact, asking a client to share their thoughts verbally too often can *impede* progress when they are in the midst of processing. Both the therapist *and* the client have to be ok with saying, 'I'm not totally sure how it worked but it did.' The goal of EMDR is to allow people to live healthy and whole in the present and the future. Regardless of what they can cognitively share from their past."

However, like all good things, EMDR isn't without its cautionary tales. Lisa warns, "Standardized EMDR Therapy and techniques are for simple traumas only. You cannot simplify complex trauma. A therapist must be trained in the complex, including attachment disorders and developmental trauma. It is important for the EMDR therapist to know how to

equip each client so that they can stay emotionally stable, and contain any traumatic material that is not currently being processed. Clients with complex trauma need to be monitored and the trauma work needs to be paced. We do not want these clients to become overwhelmed, which may push them outside their current window of tolerance."

"Unfortunately, the risk of negative reactions can be high if the therapist is unskilled or untrained to work with this population. Resulting in feelings of being overwhelmed, anxiety/panic, dissociation, and the like."

(NOTE: "Containment and resourcing" are words used to describe the skills taught by qualified, trauma-informed EMDR Practitioners to teach clients to deal with disturbing and/or unexpected memories that arise, dissociation, feelings of being overwhelmed or anxiety/panic attacks and the like.)

If you are thinking that EMDR might be right for you, make sure to ask the tough questions of your therapist. Things like, "What if I have large gaps in my story or have no event tied to my distressing emotions?" "Do you work from a developmental approach?" "How will we work on making sure I can handle what comes up? Can you teach me resources for that?" etc.

Be your own advocate. (P.S. That is a great way to provide yourself with an Emotionally Corrective Experience!)

DBT

There are times in life that we learn something new and think "where has this been all my life?!" For several of my clients, and in some ways, even for myself, DBT is exactly that. DBT stands for Dialectical Behavioral Therapy. There are four modules in standard DBT: Mindfulness, Distress Tolerance, Emotion Regulation and Interpersonal Effectiveness.

As you can tell by the names of the modules, these are skills which we can all benefit from! Consequently, they are the type of skills that would have us asking the above question: "where has this been all my life?"

In some ways, DBT is like a life skills course on steroids. Because of its practical, skill-based nature, it is a great complement to other forms of therapy, particularly therapies like EMDR, where developing resources for regulating our emotions and dealing with distressing memories are key when processing through trauma.

Having facilitated DBT therapy myself, I appreciate both the individual and group elements of the therapy, effectively mimicking the way we are designed to do life from a relational perspective. The elements of DBT also include phone coaching to help select and execute skills when you feel stuck.

A word of caution: If you Google DBT, you are going to find a lot of information about DBT and its relationship to things like personality disorders, such as Borderline Personality Disorder. Please, do *not* let that deter you or cause you to dismiss DBT as an option for your therapy.

Those articles are most prevalent because when the creator of DBT, Marsha Linehan, put these tools together, these were the people she had in mind. In fact, she developed DBT because of her own journey to healing. (Sidenote: I highly recommend her memoir *Building a Life Worth Living*.)

However, what we have discovered in the decades since its creation is that DBT has significant benefits for people struggling with addiction, relational difficulties, attachment wounds, depression and anxiety, as well as those who suffered developmental trauma.

Many of us with developmental traumas either didn't get what we needed while we were growing up, or had our emotional development

interrupted by trauma. Consequently, our ability to receive or grasp life skills to be emotionally regulated, relationally effective individuals was stunted. For those of us who did not learn these invaluable skills as children or adolescents, DBT can help fill those deficits.

In fact, for the past several years, some modules of DBT have been used in schools to help kids achieve emotional and relational success. Research shows that growth in those areas benefits them academically as well.

For further exploration, I interviewed Marianne Burke, a licensed therapist in St. Louis, Missouri, who has been practicing DBT along with EMDR for quite some time. She is an educator and lecturer in the field of DBT and facilitates a unique DBT Group for individuals who are caregivers to family members struggling with a mental illness.

I thought it might be helpful to hear from her, particularly regarding how she has seen the expansion of DBT diversify.

"It's interesting," she says with a smile. "The comment I hear consistently across the board from clients in all walks of life is 'why didn't my parents teach me this?' or 'why don't they teach this in schools?' These skills are for everyone. I'm even using DBT with couples and having tremendous success."

Marianne also sings the praises of DBT as it relates to helping people work through trauma, particularly when paired with EMDR. "The combination of DBT and EMDR for complex and extreme trauma is strong. DBT gives the client resources to not only help them stay in their window of tolerance (what we are readily capable of dealing with, emotionally speaking), but also helps them widen their window. It allows a person to learn how to stabilize themselves, so they effectively make it through the processing during EMDR."

If someone is considering DBT for themselves, Marianne has some advice. "For those who have complex trauma and struggle with regulation, I advise finding a skilled DBT therapist, trained and equipped by certified DBT trainers. They themselves should be part of a consultation team and offer group and individual therapy along with phone coaching and require diary cards from their clients."

It is important to find the right DBT group and therapist for you. If you are interested in combining DBT *with* your spirituality, you might be surprised to find how well they fit together. In my adapted DBT groups, we often referred to Scripture and writings by individuals like Henri Nouwen (in particular, his book *The Inner Voice of Love*) for our inspiration and as a starting point for our mindfulness and meditations. Scriptures like Isaiah 26:3, *"You keep him in perfect peace whose mind is stayed on you, because he trusts in you,"* speak to the mind-full-ness aspect of DBT. I say "mind-full" because incorporating the Christian perspective in DBT means we fill our minds with healthy and helpful truths from God's word *in addition to* learning how to be completely present in the moment.

Still other verses like 1 Corinthians 4:3-5 from The Message, which says *"I care very little if I am judged by you or by any human court; indeed, I do not even judge myself. 4My conscience is clear, but that does not make me innocent. It is the Lord who judges me. 5Therefore judge nothing before the appointed time; wait until the Lord comes. He will bring to light what is hidden in darkness and will expose the motives of the heart. At that time each will receive their praise from God,"* speaks rather clearly to concepts found within DBT, like a concept called Non-Judgmental Stance.

It is fairly easy to find a variety of Scripture passages that speak to how we are meant to relate with one another and create emotion regulation in our lives.

I think you will find DBT honors all aspects of how we are created and can provide incredible skills for living a healthy and full life.

IFS

The more I learn about Internal Family Systems (IFS), the more I find it to be one the most honoring therapies, in that it recognizes all parts of a person. It encourages us to explore and embrace all parts of ourselves in order to become healthy and whole.

One thing I find so interesting is that, unbeknownst to me, I have been incorporating portions of IFS in my own journey and in the work I do with clients, long before I knew what it was formally called (you can revisit an example of this in my own story).

Internal Family Systems, developed by Dr. Richard Schwartz, is an approach to therapy that combines systems thinking with the view that the mind is made up of relatively discrete subpersonalities, each with its own viewpoint and qualities. Typically, these subpersonalities (referred to as "parts") relate to some part of us in our past.

These include wounded and suppressed parts called exiles (like anger caused by the trauma we don't deal with), protective parts called managers (think in terms of the emotions we suppress from those traumatic experiences), and other protective parts called firefighters (think in terms of things like addiction or other behaviors that keep us from feeling pain). Firefighters kick in when our exiled parts show up demanding to be acknowledged.

One way to think about this in simpler terms would be to see the exile parts as our "lost child or banished adolescent," our manager parts as our "control and order" and our firefighter parts as "distractors (fun and excitement)." It is important not to label any of these parts as "bad." The

goal is to acknowledge and embrace these parts, and eventually, help guide their actions into healthier expressions that contribute to us living our best life.

This can be a bigger challenge than what we might first imagine because often, we do not like these parts of ourselves, especially our exiled parts. For those of us with childhood trauma, this can result in a reinjuring of those younger parts of ourselves we have tried to bury. We want to let these parts be seen and known. Accepted and loved. This was a big part of my story and consequently, my healing.

Some clients have said that, at first glance, they were unsure of IFS because it felt a little like saying they had multiple personalities. And, when talking about "subpersonalities" and "parts," I can see why that might be a concern. Try this: how often have you said things like "there was a part of me that wouldn't let me ...." Or "For some reason there is a part of me that doesn't trust this...." Well, in a manner of speaking, *those* are the "parts" IFS may address.

Our exiled parts, managers and firefighters, all want to protect us while simultaneously wanting us to get what we need. It's just that the means by which they try to accomplish this are often in direct contradiction to the healthy and whole life we truly want. The work of understanding and even honoring these parts, then redirecting them in their efforts is critical to creating an internal life where all parts of ourselves are working toward the same goal.

IFS is another therapy that works well with being a follower of Jesus. It isn't lost on me that Richard Schwartz, when speaking about how we can live from a place of internal integration, refers to this as "listening to our advocate." As Christians, this "advocate" is the Holy Spirit—God within us.

In her book *Boundaries for Your Soul,* Dr. Alison Cook refers to this as our "Spirit-led self." Dr. Cook states "In one of his letters, Paul wrote, 'For I delight in the law of God, in my inner being.' (Romans 7:22) These words *inner being* describe who you are at your core: your Holy Spirit-led self...."

God has designed us to live this integrated life, led by His Spirit. IFS can be a tool to help us achieve that. If you would like to explore this more, I highly recommend Dr. Cook's book. It is easy to understand and offers many stories for reflection which can help you think about how IFS can work in your life.

FINDING THE RIGHT COUNSELOR

I believe good therapy should feel like a collaboration, not an uncomfortable hierarchy.

Remember, this is a *relationship,* so it stands to reason that sometimes it will feel uncomfortable and awkward—especially in the beginning. If trust has been difficult for you, building it with your therapist and having faith in them may be difficult. It will take time. So, give yourself permission to take it at the pace you need to take.

Don't feel rushed to tell your story, especially if there is trauma. If questions are coming at you too fast or you need things to slow down, say it. Building a safe relationship before the deeper work begins should be important to both you and the therapist. However, do not use that as an excuse to avoid doing the work when the time is right. And sometimes, you might need to trust your therapist to help you see when that time is.

Having said that, be mindful that there is a difference between *processing* painful events of your past and *rehearsing* them. Telling the same stories of trauma over and over again can be like retraumatizing

yourself. We don't want to reinforce our traumatic experiences. This can heighten painful emotions and cause dysregulation.

Finally, as much as I hate to say it, if you always walk out of therapy feeling "better," then perhaps therapy is not doing what it's supposed to. Growth and healing are complicated and messy and the process feels like crap a lot of the time. Feeling some of the harder feelings is a *good* thing.

If faith is important to you, it will be most beneficial to find someone who shares in your faith, or who at least is comfortable incorporating it into your therapy. If you are a deeply religious person (this *is* different than being a deeply *spiritual* person), I would encourage you not to emphasize a therapist's religious preference over their ability to help you clinically. While it may be difficult to recognize in ourselves, some people can over-emphasize religion, or spirituality, to the detriment of their emotional, mental and even physical health. (If you're struggling here, consider going back and re-reading the *Jesus and a Therapist* section.)

By the way, we can make the same over-emphasizing mistake in other areas, too. If we lean toward more cognitive approaches, we are going to do our level best to find our answers by simply using our minds. If we are more emotional people, we can look for all the direction and the answers to be found in our feelings.

We can even take the physical too far, engaging in over-emphasizing appearance, or level of fitness of competitiveness to make us feel better, ignoring all other facets of our created being.

YOUR TURN: Reflect. Engage. Write.

Take a moment and journal about which of the therapies discussed in this section resonated with you and why.

Which of the therapies discussed do you have questions about?

What is holding you back from seeking out a therapist to walk your journey with you? How can you overcome this? Who can you ask to help you?

Write out a commitment to engage with a therapist and explore any of these therapies that you feel might be beneficial, along with other therapies recommended by a trusted, mental health professional.

The kindest approach we can take to our healing is one that embraces each area of ourselves, one that honors our mental, physical, emotional, and spiritual condition. In part, this is what being an integrated person means.

NOTE: Sometimes the first step toward our healing journey is talking through our story with someone we can trust. This might be a friend, family member, mentor or pastor. I want to encourage you to do this. Maybe consider asking them to read this book with you and share some of your responses in the ***Your Turn*** *sections. And as you think through who you might want to share your experiences with, I want to encourage you to choose someone who has proven themselves to be trustworthy. Someone whose character displays a healthy mindset and good boundaries. If possible, consider someone who has pursued their own healing and growth and reflects that in their own life. Take care to be selective in who you allow to hear your story, and who gets to speak into your life.*

THE FAITH AND SCIENCE OF GENERATIONAL IMPACT

As we draw nearer to the close of our time together, I want to revisit something from the very beginning of this book. I want to end by revisiting our mission of uncovering generational patterns, and what faith and science have to say about it.

In my research on the subject, I met Dr. Isabelle Mansuy, professor of Neuro-epigenetics at the University Zürich, Switzerland, an expert in the field of Transgenerational Epigenetic Inheritance.

One of the many fascinating things she shared in relation to how trauma is passed through generations was regarding the ability to reverse the trauma.

Dr. Mansuy shares that, "When examining the offspring from mice who had experienced trauma, their pups (who did not experience trauma first-hand) showed symptoms as they matured that mimicked symptoms as though they endured the trauma themselves."

In other words, the way the pups reacted negatively to that particular element in their environment was the result of what "carried over" from their parents, *not* because of any first-hand experience of the trauma. *The pup's reaction was based on the experiences of the generation before them.*

Dr. Mansuy goes on to say that without intervention, these symptoms are "routinely exhibited in the pups to the third and even fourth generation before symptoms begin to naturally dissipate." She states, "This seems to be consistent with what we see in humans as well." But *with* intervention, the symptoms are not only reversed in the present generation, but the future generations tend to be born with little to no remaining trauma responses related to those of the previous generations, providing there is no significant trauma reintroduced.

The implication? While trauma can impact us at a cellular level, so can healing.

In the Bible, we see countless examples of generational impact set off by the choices and behaviors of previous generations. From disconnection with God, to war, to deception and abuse, to the dangers of playing favorites amongst their children, there is no shortage of stories where we can clearly see the fall out experienced by one generation as the result of the generation(s) that went before them. We don't have room to look at details here, but you can read many of these stories in the Old Testament: 1st and 2nd Kings and/or Genesis.

Whether we are talking about science or the Bible, the consensus seems to be clear: knowing what has impacted us is critical for effecting change. When we don't know what we don't know, it can make it difficult to recognize what is necessary to experience the freedom for which we were created.

> Healing our wounds is like building a dam to protect the generations that come after us. It is like telling the traumatic rapids of our past, "You cannot rage beyond this point."

ENDINGS AND BEGINNINGS

Well, my Brave Friend, we have certainly covered a lot of territory together! Thank you for sticking it out and completing this journey with me, even when the road got bumpy.

I am honored you trusted me enough to read what I've shared and am excited for what this book may have inspired you to pursue.

As I sit and type this last handful of words, I am already praying that whenever you read them, it is with new insights and a deeper sense of hope. I pray that this book has helped you find the courage to explore your story and the stories of those who went before you.

It would be my greatest joy to know that this journey has emboldened you to pursue the resources you need to create your best life. Lastly, I pray that you have found your true voice. May this be your first step toward breaking cycles, slaying shame, and finding freedom, for yourself and for the generations to come.

PART ELEVEN

Epilogue

"If we don't transform our pain, we are certain to transmit it."
RICHARD ROHR

Dear Friend,

A few days ago (from the time when I am writing this), I completed ***Generations Deep*** and passed it on to the hands of a dear friend (a writer herself) who so graciously volunteered to read it through to help ensure my thoughts and ideas make sense to more than just me.

It was difficult to let it go, as that meant trusting I have written down the words that need to be here and left out the ones that didn't.

When my writer-friend finishes with it, the words on these pages will pass to another, and another, each person carefully selected for their talents and hearts for this project. As the pages pass from person to person, it will be gently cleaned up and aligned along the way, fixing the mishaps and mistakes until it eventually becomes this book you hold in your hands.

But today, the moment my brain came online, even before my eyes greeted the dawn, a thought was loudly playing over in my mind. One that basically demanded to be shared with you. And so, this epilogue was born.

I hope your time with me here has offered something valuable and good for your life. If you ever want to share your experiences, I would love to hear them.

Wait! That's not the compelling thought. This is...

Among the things you walk away with from your time in this book, there is one thing I want to make sure you hear *very* clearly. Just as recognizing the generational patterns in your family doesn't doom you to repeat them, understanding them and calling them out into the light alone won't break them.

Remember, knowledge is only power when its combined with action.

Use any revelation or work you have done while reading this book, anything you have learned here, experienced here, as your foundation for the deeper work. Use it to help you see how God fits in to your journey. Use it to help you heal, to break cycles and slay shame. Use it to help you find the freedom you were created for. But don't do it alone.

Oh, and listen carefully. Can you hear it? That's the sound of me, cheering you on.

"Christ has set us free to live a free life.
So, take your stand!"
Galatians 5:1 MSG

IT TAKES A VILLAGE

One of my favorite verses in the Bible is Proverbs 27:17. In the Message translation, it says, *"Steel sharpens steel. And one friend sharpens another."*

I am incredibly grateful for the friends I have been blessed with who sharpen me where I am dull, and smooth out my edges where I am rough and sharp.

This book could not have possibly become all it was intended to be without the wisdom of these friends and colleagues whom God has so graciously placed in my life... and *always* at the right time.

Before we get to the list of incredible humans who have helped make ***Generations Deep*** the book that it is, I want to express my deepest love and gratitude for my husband, Tom. Sadly, words are just too limiting to describe how supportive and encouraging he has been. He is my greatest love and, as I said at the beginning of the book, my greatest emotionally corrective experience.

To my kiddos by blood, Ariel and Alexander, and to my bonus kiddos, Sam, Alex, Ben, I want you to know that you all are the reason(s) I continued on the journey to healing. You're also the reason I refuse to settle where I am now, and not only continue to seek more growth for myself, but to pass on whatever I learn to others. Especially to each of you. It is the prayer of my heart to be for each of you what I missed in my own life. I love you all so much.

To my sisters from other misters, Chrissy and Julie. Thank you for being my family when I had none. Thank you for cheering me on and for loving my special kind of crazy. Julie, you were the first to say, "you should write a book about your story." And Chrissy, you were the first one to read it! Typos and all! (SO many typos!) Thank you for praying for me,

for holding up my arms when I couldn't hold them up for myself and for being the kind of sisters a girl longs for.

When I first began to work on this project, I was privileged to have the wise counsel and friendship of Ginger Moran, PhD. Her guidance helped me in the formative portions of this book and to her I owe a great debt of gratitude.

As the book progressed, I recognized the need for a doula, if you will. Someone to coach me through the hard labor and delivery of ***Generations Deep***. I found that and more in book coach extraordinaire, Michelle Cox. Michelle has talked me off several ledges and given me the good and sometimes hard truth needed to bring this project into the world. Michelle, you are a force to be reckoned with. I am grateful for your expertise and your friendship.

I am deeply indebted to all the counselors who have contributed to this book, whether in sharing their personal stories with me or contributing to the **Expanded Trauma Perspective Questionnaire**. In particular, a special thank you to David Koch LPC, who helped me put the questionnaire together.

To the Beta Team who gave *the most* detailed, genuine, challenging and helpful feedback an author could ask for. Elizabeth, Mandy, Christi, Tiffany, Jeff, Sandra, Erin, Michele, Sandy, Catherine, Polly, Erin, Caitlin, Anna and Dondra, your contributions are an invaluable gift to me. ***Generations Deep*** is richer and fuller because of you and for that I will be eternally grateful.

And speaking of a richer and fuller result, I am super grateful for Kate Hodel, editor and finder of all things squirrely. Sidenote: remember the "other offer on the lake home?" Well, guess what? That was Kate (and her awesome hubby, Tony). God knew we needed to be friends, so, while we were the ones who got *our* lake home, Kate and Tony ended

up getting a home just two doors down from us! When she heard about this project she was adamant that she become the editor and I would have been foolish to turn her down. Kate, thank you for the gift of your mad skills and beautiful friendship.

Finally, my greatest debt of gratitude is to my Jesus. You saved me. You wired me in such a way that the therapy I experienced was able to work. You didn't give up on me. You helped me heal. And you gave me everything and every relationship that has made my life better and made this book better, too. My prayer is that the work I do will reflect Your heart for people, and the freedom that only You can provide.

You indeed, Jesus, make all things new.

For more information on the resources mentioned in ***Generations Deep***, or for additional resources to help you heal and grow, visit **www.itsmyoutloudvoice.com/resources**.

For bonus resources and content, visit **www.generationsdeep.com**.

For more information on EMDR or to find an EMDR therapist in your area, go to **www.emdria.org/find-a-therapist**.

For more information on IFS or to find an IFS Practitioner, go to **www.ifs-institute.com/practitioners**.

For more information on DBT or to find a DBT Therapist, go to **www.behavioraltech.org/resources/find-a-therapist**.

If you wish to contact Gina, you can email her directly at **gina@itsmyoutloudvoice.com**.

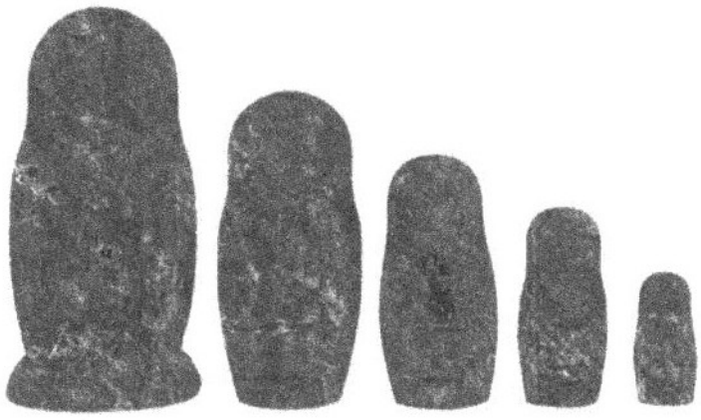

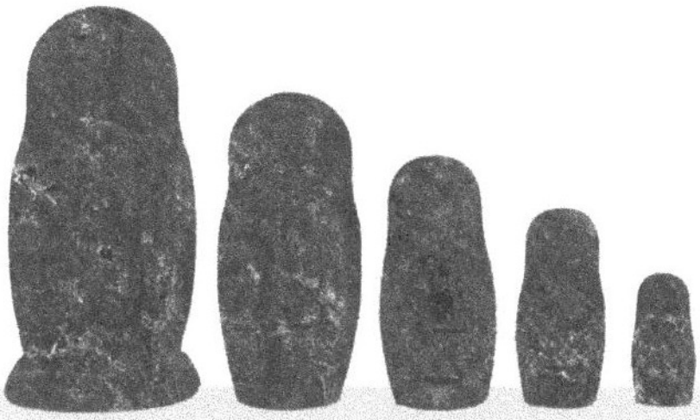

Generations/Family Relationships Chart

Name (Relative)	Biological Relationship	Adopted Relationship	Step Relationship
Lucia/Lucy	Great-grandmother	Great-grandmother*	
Julie	Great-aunt	Grandmother*	
Albert	Great-uncle	Great-uncle*	
Antonio/Tony	Great-grandfather	Great-grandfather*	
Marie	Grandmother	Great-aunt**	
Charlie	Grandfather	N/A (Absent)**	
Cathy	Mother	Cousin*+	
Dean	Father	N/A (absent)*^	
Dave			Stepfather
Judy	Cousin	Mother	
Ernie		Father	
Corky	Cousin	Uncle	
Katie	Cousin	N/A (absent)**	

** *Completely absent from my life growing up.*

* *Known to me only briefly.*

*+ *Cathy was not known to me until Julie's funeral.*

*^ *Dean was not a part of my life until 2017.*

Made in USA - Kendallville, IN
85318_9781732954526
02.04.2022 1420